CLINICAL NURSE SPECIALIST TOOLKIT

Melanie Duffy, MSN, RN, CCRN, CCNS, is a clinical nurse specialist (CNS) in critical care at Pinnacle Health System, Harrisburg, Pennsylvania, and adjunct faculty at Widener University, Chester, Pennsylvania. She is a past president of the National Association of Clinical Nurse Specialists (NACNS) and cochairs the Legislative/Regulatory Committee of NACNS. She is a member of other professional organizations including the American Association of Critical-Care Nurses (AACN), Sigma Theta Tau, and the American Nurses Association (ANA). Her professional influence has been in promoting the role, practice, and leadership aspects of the CNS. She has been an active presenter at national, state, and local meetings. Ms. Duffy was actively involved in gaining title recognition in Pennsylvania for the CNS and is currently working on legislation to implement a scope of practice for the CNS in Pennsylvania.

Susan Dresser, MSN, RN, APRN-CNS, CCRN, currently teaches in the clinical nurse specialist (CNS) program at the University of Oklahoma College of Nursing in Oklahoma City. She is a past secretary and board member of the National Association of Clinical Nurse Specialists (NACNS) and a past president of the Oklahoma Association of Clinical Nurse Specialists. Ms. Dresser is an active member of the American Association of Critical-Care Nurses (AACN), and has served as president, secretary, and chair of the Program Committee in the Oklahoma City chapter. She has held multiple positions as a critical care and cardiovascular CNS throughout her career. She obtained her MSN in the adult critical care CNS program at Duke University and is currently enrolled in the PhD program at the University of Kansas Medical Center School of Nursing.

Janet S. Fulton, PhD, RN, ACNS-BC, ANEF, FAAN, is a professor at Indiana University School of Nursing and coordinator of the Adult/Gerontology (clinical nurse specialist [CNS]) program. She is the editor-in-chief of *Clinical Nurse Specialist: The International Journal of Advanced Nursing Practice* and past president of the National Association of Clinical Nurse Specialists (NACNS). She also served as coordinator of the Oncology Nursing Society's CNS Special Interest Group and was a member of the American Nurses Association Council of CNS. She is widely published in the area of CNS practice and education, and is coeditor of *Foundations of Clinical Nurse Specialist Practice*, the only comprehensive textbook for CNS students.

CLINICAL NURSE SPECIALIST TOOLKIT

TOOLKIT

A Guide for the New Clinical Nurse Specialist

Second Edition

Melanie Duffy, MSN, RN, CCRN, CCNS
Susan Dresser, MSN, RN, APRN-CNS, CCRN
Janet S. Fulton, PhD, RN, ACNS-BC, ANEF, FAAN
EDITORS

Co-Published With the
National Association of Clinical Nurse Specialists (NACNS)

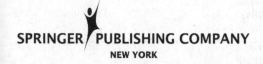

SPRINGER PUBLISHING COMPANY
NEW YORK

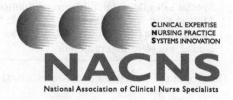

CLINICAL EXPERTISE
NURSING PRACTICE
SYSTEMS INNOVATION

NACNS
National Association of Clinical Nurse Specialists

Springer Publishing Company, LLC
11 West 42nd Street
New York, NY 10036
www.springerpub.com

Acquisitions Editor: Margaret Zuccarini
Composition: diacriTech

ISBN: 978-0-8261-7191-7
e-book ISBN: 978-0-8261-7192-4

16 17 18 19/ 5 4 3 2 1

The author and the publisher of this Work have made every effort to use sources believed to be reliable to provide information that is accurate and compatible with the standards generally accepted at the time of publication. The author and publisher shall not be liable for any special, consequential, or exemplary damages resulting, in whole or in part, from the readers' use of, or reliance on, the information contained in this book. The publisher has no responsibility for the persistence or accuracy of URLs for external or third-party Internet websites referred to in this publication and does not guarantee that any content on such websites is, or will remain, accurate or appropriate.

Library of Congress Cataloging-in-Publication Data
Names: Duffy, Melanie, editor. | Dresser, Susan, editor. | Fulton, Janet S.,
    editor. | National Association of Clinical Nurse Specialists.
Title: Clinical nurse specialist toolkit : a guide for the new clinical nurse
    specialist / Melanie Duffy, MSN, RN, CCRN, CCNS, Susan Dresser, MSN, RN,
    APRN-BC, CCRN, Janet S. Fulton, PhD, RN, ACNS-BC, ANEF, FAAN, editors.
Description: Second edition. | New York, NY : Springer Publishing Company,
    LLC, [2016] | "Co-Published with the National Association of Clinical
    Nurse Specialists (NACNS)." | Includes bibliographical references and
    index.
Identifiers: LCCN 2015044641 | ISBN 9780826171917
Subjects: LCSH: Nurse practitioners.
Classification: LCC RT82.8 .C576 2016 | DDC 610.7306/92--dc23 LC record available at
http://lccn.loc.gov/2015044641

Printed in the United States of America by Gasch Printing.

This book is dedicated to clinical nurse specialists (CNSs) everywhere—those currently practicing in the role, those using CNS knowledge and abilities in other roles, and those no longer in active practice. Once a CNS, always a CNS!

Contents

Contributors   xi
Preface   xv

Part I Getting Started

1. Negotiating a Job   3
   Christine Schulman

2. Creating a Job Description   13
   Kathleen M. Vollman, Denise O'Brien, and Cathy C. Lewis

3. Finding a Place in the Organization   23
   Jan Powers

4. Working With "The Boss"   33
   Ann M. Herbage Busch

Part II Moving Forward

5. Learning the Ropes: Orientation   45
   Ruthann B. Zafian

6. Establishing Credibility   55
   Ruth Van Gerpen

7. Prioritizing: Avoiding Overcommitment and Underachievement   61
   Katie Brush

8. Finding a Mentor   69
   Vivian Donahue

9. Using the Internet: Guide to Internet-Based Resources   77
   Barbara Manz Friesth and Susan K. B. Jones

Part III Gaining Momentum

10. Leading Groups   *87*
    Melissa A. Lowder

11. Mentoring Staff   *97*
    Patricia A. Foster

12. Precepting Students   *105*
    Ginger S. Pierson

13. Championing Evidence-Based Practice   *115*
    Deborah J. Schafer

Part IV Evaluation

14. Documenting Clinical Outcomes   *129*
    Deborah G. Klein

15. Reporting Out: Communicating to Multiple Audiences   *137*
    Melanie Duffy and Janet S. Fulton

Part V Reaching Out

16. Becoming Involved With Professional Organizations   *149*
    Mary Fran Tracy and Patrick Schultz

17. Working With Community Agencies   *157*
    Sharon D. Horner, Cara C. Young, and Karen E. Johnson

18. Networking   *169*
    Mary A. Stahl

19. Facilitating Transitions of Care   *177*
    Paula A. O'Hearn Ulch and Mary M. Schmidt

20. Participating in Interprofessional Education   *189*
    Jennifer L. Embree and Janet S. Fulton

Part VI Professional Recognition

21. Obtaining Certification: Considering the Options   *203*
    Melanie Duffy

22. Navigating the Privileging and Credentialing Process   *211*
    Susan Sendelbach

23. Qualifying for Reimbursement   *215*
    Susan Dresser

24. Starting Collaborative Practice With Physicians or Clinics: What You
Should Know   *227*
Carol L. Delville, Sheri Innerarity, and Glenda Joiner-Rogers

25. Secrets for a Joyful Life as a Clinical Nurse Specialist   *237*
Janet S. Fulton

Index   *243*

Contributors

Katie Brush, MS, RN, CCRN, CCNS, FCCM (Deceased)
Massachusetts General Hospital
Boston, Massachusetts

Ann M. Herbage Busch, MS, RN, CWOCN, ACNS-BC-PP, FAAN
Portland Veterans Administration Medical Center
Portland, Oregon

Carol L. Delville, PhD, APRN, ACNS-BC
The University of Texas at Austin School of Nursing
Austin, Texas

Vivian Donahue, MS, RN, ACNS, CCRN
Massachusetts General Hospital
Boston, Massachusetts

Susan Dresser, MSN, RN, APRN-CNS, CCRN
University of Oklahoma College of Nursing
Oklahoma City, Oklahoma

Melanie Duffy, MSN, RN, CCRN, CCNS
Pinnacle Health System
Harrisburg, Pennsylvania

Jennifer L. Embree, DNP, RN, NE-BC, CCNS
Indiana University School of Nursing
Indianapolis, Indiana

Patricia A. Foster, MS, RN, ACNS-BC, CNS, CWOCN, CMSRN (Retired)
Apache Junction, Arizona

Barbara Manz Friesth, PhD, RN
Indiana University School of Nursing
Indianapolis, Indiana

Janet S. Fulton, PhD, RN, ACNS-BC, ANEF, FAAN
Indiana State University School of Nursing
Indianapolis, Indiana

Sharon D. Horner, PhD, RN, FAAN
The University of Texas at Austin School of Nursing
Austin, Texas

Sheri Innerarity, PhD, RN, ACNS, FNP-BC
The University of Texas at Austin School of Nursing
Austin, Texas

Karen E. Johnson, PhD, RN
The University of Texas at Austin School of Nursing
Austin, Texas

Glenda Joiner-Rogers, PhD, RN, ACNS-BC
The University of Texas at Austin School of Nursing
Austin, Texas

Susan K. B. Jones, MS, RN, APN, CCNS-P, CCRN-P
INTEGRIS Health
Oklahoma City, Oklahoma

Deborah G. Klein, MSN, RN, ACNS-BC, CCRN, CHFN, FAHA
Cleveland Clinic
Cleveland, Ohio

Cathy C. Lewis, MSN, RN
University of Michigan Hospital and Health Systems
Ann Arbor, Michigan

Melissa A. Lowder, DNP, RN, ACNS-BC, CCRN
Franciscan St. Francis Hospital
Indianapolis, Indiana

Denise O'Brien, DNP, RN, ACNS-BC, CPAN, CAPA, FAAN
University of Michigan Hospital and Health Systems
Ann Arbor, Michigan

Ginger S. Pierson, MSN, RN, CCRN, CCNS
West Coast University
Anaheim, California

Jan Powers, PhD, RN, CCNS, CCRN, CNRN, FCCM
Parkview Regional Medical Center
Fort Wayne, Indiana

Deborah J. Schafer, MSN, RNC-OB, CNS
Pinnacle Health System
Harrisburg, Pennsylvania

Mary M. Schmidt, MS, RN, CNS-BC
Aurora Health Care
Milwaukee, Wisconsin

Christine Schulman, MS, RN, CNS, CCRN
Legacy Health
Portland, Oregon

Patrick Schultz, MS, RN, ACNS-BC
Sanford Medical Center Fargo
Fargo, North Dakota

Susan Sendelbach, PhD, APRN, CNS, FAHA, FAAN
Abbott Northwestern Hospital
Minneapolis, Minnesota

Mary A. Stahl, MSN, RN, ACNS-BC, CCNS-CMC, Alumnus CCRN
American Association of Critical-Care Nurses
Aliso Viejo, California

Mary Fran Tracy, PhD, RN, APRN, CNS, FAAN
University of Minnesota Medical Center
Minneapolis, Minnesota

Paula A. O'Hearn Ulch, MSN, RN, CNS-BC
Aurora Health Care
Milwaukee, Wisconsin

Ruth Van Gerpen, MS, RN-BC, APRN-CNS, AOCNS(r)
Bryan Health
Lincoln, Nebraska

Kathleen M. Vollman, MSN, RN, CCNS, FCCM, FAAN
Advancing Nursing, LLC
Northville, Michigan

Cara C. Young, PhD, RN, FNP-C
The University of Texas at Austin School of Nursing
Austin, Texas

Ruthann B. Zafian, MSN, MA, ACNS-BC, APRN
Hartford Hospital
Hartford, Connecticut

Preface

This book was initially conceived about 10 years ago by clinical nurse specialists (CNSs) serving on the National Association of Clinical Nurse Specialists (NACNS) Board of Directors. While informally sharing stories of those early years of CNS practice, it became evident that the wisdom embedded in the stories of experienced CNSs should be made available to new CNSs as they begin their professional journey. Regardless of specialty or setting, transitioning to CNS practice brings similar challenges. Experienced CNSs should help ease the way for those following behind. Hence, this book was initially intended as a collection of practical tips and helpful information written by experienced CNSs as advice to new CNSs.

This new edition continues in the tradition of the initial work. It is designed for a new CNS, as well as the more experienced CNS looking for some advice and new ideas. We retained the idea of a toolkit because of the focus on practical guidance for success. Our contributing authors share lessons learned, personal insights, and proven strategies for succeeding in the CNS role from the perspective of experience.

Building on the success of the first edition, this second edition contains updated information and new material addressing current challenges in health care issues faced by CNSs. There is new content addressing evidence-based practice, interprofessional education, and managing a research study or clinical project. And because CNS practice is expanding to new settings with new practice configurations, there is new content on working in outpatient settings and collaborating with physicians in primary care. CNS practice is multifaceted, occurs in the three well-recognized domains of patient/client, nurses/nursing practice and organizations/systems, and serves as a voice of advanced nursing at the bedside and in the boardroom. This toolkit offers advice for success across that broad range of CNS practice.

As editors, we thank our author contributors for sharing their expertise and personal stories—they made this book the best possible! And we thank our publisher, Margaret Zuccarini at Springer Publishing Company, for her steadfast guidance and patience. And to CNSs everywhere, we wish each of you a long and joyful career as a CNS!

Melanie Duffy
Susan Dresser
Janet S. Fulton

PART I
GETTING STARTED

CHAPTER 1

Negotiating a Job

CHRISTINE SCHULMAN

The dream job for any clinical nurse specialist (CNS) is one that will be satisfying and challenging over time. Negotiating the fine details to make that happen is an ongoing process that starts at the time of hire and extends throughout the time you have the position. First things first, however: You must successfully navigate several phases of the job search process before you will negotiate the details of an exciting offer. Being clear on what you enjoy about your work, about the job you are being offered, and about what you personally need to be successful are essential for making an educated decision about your work. This chapter first focuses on reflecting about what you enjoy about being a CNS and then preparing for the job search. Next, it provides suggestions for a powerful and insightful interview with a prospective employer, colleagues, and clients. Finally, key points to negotiate before accepting the job offer, along with specific items to address, are discussed. A successful journey along these steps will help you identify and get the job that will create and sustain your professional enthusiasm over the long haul.

PREPARING FOR THE JOB SEARCH

Preparatory work for the interview is critical to making a good impression with your prospective employer as well as making sure you get the information you need to make an informed decision about the position. This includes thinking about your role as a CNS, developing your professional portfolio, identifying life issues that influence your ability to meet the job requirements, and researching the institution where you seek employment.

Reflect on Your Role as a CNS

Spend time preparing for the interview process by reflecting on your vision of the CNS role, your interests and talents, and your personal life issues that must be considered when applying for a position. Thinking about these things is important to ensure a good match between what you want and the actual job. Once you've identified these issues, be watchful for how they are addressed throughout the entire application process, beginning with the first interview until the time when you are offered the position.

Ask yourself the following questions: Why did I become a CNS? Which of the main components of the role (education and mentoring, quality improvement, protocol development, research) give me the most satisfaction? How do my skills align with the components of the role? Are my passions in alignment with the job requirements? What does the "perfect CNS day" look like? Answers to these questions provide structure for discussion during your interviews. Alignment of these important issues with what you've discovered about the job during the application process will influence your decision to accept or decline the job offer.

Prepare a Portfolio

You will be asked to describe your work experience. While a curriculum vitae (CV) or résumé presents an excellent overview of your accomplishments, it doesn't reveal how you think, communicate, and accomplish work. A portfolio will help you show interviewers not just what you have accomplished but how you work. The "oral" portfolio consists of stories illustrating your experiences with communication, conflict management, prioritization, outcomes management, financial issues, and involvement with professional organizations. If you recently completed your graduate program, you will need to emphasize group and individual school projects. Have these examples fresh in your memory and well rehearsed so that they are concise and clearly illustrate your point. The "written" portfolio includes the hard copy evidence of your work. Depending on the position for which you are applying it should include some, if not all, of the following items:

- Published journal articles or book chapters, ideally regarding your area of expertise
- Printouts of research or quality improvement (QI) posters presented at professional conferences
- A handout from one of your best presentations
- A descriptive summary of a project you led, with outcome data (if not confidential)
- A protocol, policy, or procedure that you wrote
- An evaluation summary of a class you taught or course you coordinated

Identify Important Life Issues

Life issues are as important as your education and your experience in identifying whether you are able to meet the requirements of the job. These questions often address scheduling challenges (e.g., Do you need to arrive at work after 8:00 a.m.? Are you able to work the occasional evening and night shift? Do you need flexibility in your start and stop times due to child care or other transportation issues?). Think about how much time you can give the position; the reality of the CNS role is that there are always periods when you need to put in extra time to get work done. You need to know if your home responsibilities or personal energies are such that they cannot accommodate frequent overtime so that you do not accept a position where the usual workweek exceeds 50 hours.

Research the Prospective Employer

Resources in effective interviewing consistently state the importance of researching your potential workplace (Byham & Pickett, 1999; Pohly, n.d.; U.S. Department of Labor, 2005). How big is the institution? Is it an academic or a community facility? Is it a profit, nonprofit, or government-run entity? How many of its patients are Medicare patients? What are the centers of emphasis (in order to determine if the institution's priorities are consistent with your areas of interest)? Can you get a sense of how it is responding to the Affordable Care Act? What is the institution's model for delivery of care? Is it a Magnet institution, or has it received other recognitions for excellence? What is its reputation in the nursing community? Is it unionized? Does it have a relationship with a university to support ongoing education of its employees? These questions identify the type of facility that will support your professional needs and interests over time and will also help you develop questions you should ask during your interview to explore areas of interest or concern.

Research State Licensure Requirements

The anticipated date for full implementation of the Advanced Practice Registered Nursing (APRN) Consensus Model is late 2015. (American Nurses Credentialing Center, 2015; National Council of State Boards of Nursing, 2010). This model, completed in 2008, will enable APRNs to consistently practice to the full extent of their education and licensure. It will provide much needed consistency between the different state requirements for licensure, certification, accreditation, and education. To date, variability among states still exists and creates challenges for candidates who wish to relocate to a different state for employment. Some states may have grandfather clauses, allowing candidates who have previously functioned in the CNS role to qualify for licensure even though they are not certified or their academic program did not include the required 500 clinical hours or "3 Ps" courses (physiology, pharmacology, and physical assessment). But many states do not have grandfather clauses or their clauses have expired. Moving forward, state boards of nursing and certification organizations will consider only APRN candidates who have completed the requirements (Hartigan, 2011).

Research the APRN regulations for the state where you hope to relocate. Explore what certification exams are required for the role you seek. Determine whether the CNS falls within the APRN definition for that particular state or whether there is separate title protection and licensure. By researching these issues in advance of your interview, you can prevent the disappointing experience of being accepted for a position in a state that may be unable to grant you a license.

PREPARING FOR THE INTERVIEW

A full discussion of how to have an effective job interview is beyond the scope of this chapter; however, there are numerous, excellent resources available to help you prepare (Block & Petrus, 2004; Byham & Pickett, 1999; Fitzwater, 2001; Kessler, 2006; Powers, 2000; Welton, Morton, & Amig, 1998). The following discussion focuses on the elements that will help you identify key issues that usually surface during the final negotiations of a CNS position.

You should develop responses to questions that are likely to be asked. Some questions will be simple and direct, such as: What is appealing to you about being a CNS? Are you able to work the night shift? What training do you have in data analysis? How do you communicate to others that you are stressed? Many employers use "behavioral interviews" by asking open-ended questions that allow you to describe real events and your role in them. The interviewer is looking for you to describe in detail your role in a particular event, project, or experience and what the outcome was (Fitzwater, 2001; Pohly, n.d.; Quintessential Careers, n.d.). Hearing about your past performance can help prospective employers predict your future performance in similar circumstances. Their objective is to identify your communication skills, your prioritization of work demands, your ability to resolve conflict, your clinical expertise, and your ability to navigate change. Use examples from school, internships, previous jobs, and volunteer work. Highlight special professional and personal accomplishments such as the money raised from a professional conference that you coordinated or the marathon that you finished within your expected time frame. The examples you choose should demonstrate critical thinking abilities, motivation and self-leadership, a willingness to learn and be creative, an ability to work as part of a team, professionalism, and self-confidence (Hansens, n.d.). Behavioral questions may also try to identify your response to negative situations and how you learned from them (Quintessential Careers, n.d.).

To prepare for behavior-based interviews, think about several examples where you demonstrated excellent performance in areas in which the employer will be interested: Clinical issues, team building, change management, and conflict resolution are commonly explored during interviews. You should also be prepared to describe situations that started out negatively but ended positively because you either made the best of the outcome or learned from that experience to behave differently the next time a similar situation arose. Make sure that your examples illustrate a variety of experiences from your work and professional life. Rehearse telling these stories so that you quickly get to the point and do not wander off topic; every story should have a clear beginning, middle, and end. Examples of topics likely to surface during your interview can be found in Table 1.1.

Use the STAR format to structure concise answers to behavioral questions (Quintessential Careers, n.d.).

- **Situation or Task**: Specifically describe the situation you were in or the task you needed to accomplish. Give enough detail for the interviewer to understand, but not so much that you wander off track or lose the attention of the interviewer.

TABLE 1.1 Behavioral Interview Topics for the CNS Candidate

- Describe how you implemented new research findings into practice at your institution.
- Tell about an incident where you formed and developed a team.
- Describe how you resolved a conflict with a supervisor, colleague, or client.
- Describe how you identified and managed a need within your institution.
- Give an example of when you had to share difficult feedback.
- Describe a quality or process improvement project that you coordinated.
- Tell about how you set and achieved a personal or professional goal.
- Describe the most difficult project you have ever tackled. Describe the outcome, and what you learned from the experience.
- Tell about a time when you had to partner with someone whose work style was very different from yours.
- Give an example of a good (or bad) decision that you made and what you learned from that decision.
- Tell about a situation when you had to build consensus within a group of diverse people.
- Give an example of how you prioritized multiple demands. How did you manage your stress during this time?
- Describe a time when you had to communicate information or a practice change that was unpopular. How did you approach it? Did you achieve buy-in? What was the result?
- Describe a situation in which you had to support an administrative decision with which you personally did not agree. How did you do this? How did you reconcile this to yourself?
- Describe a project in which you had to maintain tight fiscal control. Did you accomplish your financial goals?
- Describe your management style. Give examples of when this has been helpful and when it has been a handicap.

- **Action:** Describe the action you took. Keep the focus of the story on your role and activities, even if describing a team project. Tell what you actually did, not what you should have done.
- **Results:** Describe the outcome of the event. Were goals accomplished? What were the lessons learned?

An interview is a two-way street, so you must also plan to ask questions. Asking good questions will provide you with the information you need, and it will also demonstrate to your interviewer your critical thinking abilities and priorities (Block & Petrus, 2004; Career Consulting Corner, n.d.). This is not the time to ask about salary or work hours; this is the time to ask about relationships, priorities, and work processes at the institution in which you seek employment. Use the principles of behavioral interviews already described to encourage the interviewer to answer your questions with clear examples. Ask interviewers to provide examples of how a CNS led a specific project, how the organization responded to a CNS's recommendation for a practice change, or how the supervisor helped a CNS make decisions about competing priorities. Failure to take advantage of this opportunity to question the interviewer could result in unpleasant surprises later and may suggest to the interviewer that your level of interest and commitment to the job may be limited.

All interviewers and interview panels should be asked to share their vision of the CNS role at the institution. They should also be asked to describe how past key projects have been prioritized, to identify initial needs that must be addressed, to describe the orientation plan and evaluation criteria, to clarify the reporting structure, to address the working style of the team, and to address a typical workday or workweek. Get clarification about who you will report to: Will this person be a nursing administrator, a hospital administrator, or a unit nurse manager? Ask to see the organizational structure of the facility and of the nursing division so you can assess the power of nursing within that institution and the "political" climate. It is important to inquire about support for professional development opportunities (e.g., participation in professional organizations, writing for publication, presentations at national conferences, affiliations with industry).

Ask your prospective employer to clarify the scope of the job. How does the facility differentiate the CNS role and its responsibilities from those of the nurse manager, nurse educator, or coordinator of nursing quality? Will you be responsible for a geographical clinical area or a specific patient population throughout the hospital (e.g., the sixth floor telemetry unit or all cardiology patients in the facility from emergency department admission to cardiac rehabilitation)? Will you have responsibilities on several campuses within that hospital system? Will you be required to do direct patient care? If so, under what circumstances might this happen? Will you have responsibilities outside of your immediate clinical area (e.g., chair of the hospital-wide pain committee, tracking and reporting central line and surgical site infection data within the system and nationally)? CNS and educator colleagues should be asked how they distribute the workload and communicate with one another. Ask for examples of how the supervisor advocated for him or her when there were multiple demands for the CNS's time. Similarities or differences in answers will suggest the degree to which the team communicates and perceives the work environment.

Preparing to have an effective interview is of paramount importance as it provides the potential employer the opportunity to learn about you and how you will contribute to the organization. No less important, however, is that the interview allows you to learn about that institution and determine whether it is a place in which you wish to work.

NEGOTIATING THE JOB OFFER

Once you have received a job offer, you are given another opportunity to fine-tune the position to sustain your professional interests without sacrificing important lifestyle issues. This is the time to negotiate the details to foster your professional success. You are in the driver's seat. You must clarify questions from your earlier interviews, further explore areas of concern or interest, and work out the details of financial compensation, benefits, and scheduling. Advocate for yourself, but show willingness to compromise to meet the needs of the organization while not sacrificing what is important to your long-term satisfaction and performance.

The first types of questions address the basic structure of your job: when do you start, relocation reimbursement, what your work schedule will be, and, most importantly, salary and benefits. The last two items may be addressed by someone in human resources. Regardless of whom you speak with about salary, it is critical that you are familiar with the range of CNS salaries in your community. You need to know if the proposed compensation is comparable to what is available elsewhere in your region. Consider whether the salary, health care and vacation benefits, and support for professional advancement add up to a reasonable package compared with other options in your geographical area. For example, the salary might be slightly lower than the community standard, but this might be favorably balanced against something else that is particularly attractive to you, such as tuition compensation if you wish to go back to school, flexible hours if you have children who have school transportation needs, or an option for a 4-day workweek rather than the traditional 5-day workweek. It all boils down to what is important to your professional and personal needs. CNSs are "jacks of all trades" who are invaluable to an institution and, therefore, should be compensated with time, money, and professional benefits to reflect this. If the sum of these benefits is substandard, then continue to negotiate or consider declining the offer.

It is important to clarify how your work will be assigned and prioritized. Work assignments coming from more than one person can result in conflict and unreasonable demands on your time. The ultimate result of this disorganization is that you will become frustrated, miss deadlines, and produce work that is not the quality that you prefer.

If you have not yet met with your immediate peer group, ask to do so now. Here you want to ask questions to help you ascertain the collegiality of the group. In other words: Do they work and play well together? How do they distribute workload? How do they partner on projects? How do they cover for one another for illness, vacations, and holidays? Will you be part of a specific CNS group, and does participating in that group add to your responsibilities? Watch body language closely during this meeting: Is there laughter and a sense of cohesiveness in the group? Does anyone stand out as being different from the group or different from you, such that he or she might be difficult to work with? Much of the work of the CNS is relationship based, so it is important that your cohort be people you enjoy, can work with, and can learn from.

The next set of questions, listed in Table 1.2, has to do with getting started in the role and ensuring that you will receive the technical support you need to do your work. Ask about the plan for your orientation and how long it will last. Be leery of any promise to find you an office after you have started or situations where you are expected to share a computer. Hospitals frequently have limited office space. It could be months before you find a place to call "home," which could adversely impact your productivity. It may be necessary to negotiate your start date based on when your office is expected to be available. There is no need to be unrealistic regarding this issue, such as demanding a private office with a window! The ideal space is one that places you either with your peer group or with the unit where you will be doing most of your work so that you are immediately accessible to the nursing staff, physicians, and your colleagues. Ask if it is permissible to work from home, especially when projects that require quiet time (e.g., writing an article) are under tight deadlines.

Another "red flag" is if there is no clerical or administrative support to help you with paperwork and routine office activities (e.g., processing course registrations, tallying course evaluations, data entry). While you are certainly able to do these activities, your time and expertise as a CNS is more appropriately

---

TABLE 1.2 Negotiating the Fine Points of the Job Offer

- Will there be an office space established on the day that you start?
- Will there be a pager, phone, computer, and so forth ready on the start date or reasonably soon thereafter?
- Is there clerical/administrative support when you need it?
- Will there be a parking space available? Will you have to pay for parking?
- How often will you be expected to leave the hospital mid-day, making having a car essential? Are there other transportation alternatives?
- Who will be your preceptor during orientation?
- How often should you meet with your supervisor during orientation?
- Who will give feedback during orientation and the first year?
- What are the priorities for the first 6 months? The first year?

spent on the clinical issues on which you were hired to work. The institution for which you want to work should have people in place so that you do not have to spend time doing clerical work. Most CNSs will say it is often easier and quicker to do something themselves because they are thinking and creating while typing the document. That being said, there needs to be support for clerical tasks so that your energies can be focused on nursing concerns. Speaking with your potential peer group about the amount of administrative support will help you identify if this is an issue you need to consider before making your decision.

THINKING IT OVER

You have spent a lot of time and energy preparing for the interview that will lead to a job offer. In response to that offer, more issues have been explored, negotiated, and agreed upon. You now have all of the information you need to make a smart decision about this professional opportunity. Your friends and colleagues will offer solicited and unsolicited advice, warnings, and encouragement. There is value in listening to their input, certainly, but it is more important to listen to yourself and your internal dialogue. Is this a job that you want to do? Do you think it will be interesting? Will you like the patients, your colleagues, and the work you will be asked to do? Has there been good dialogue with the people you have met? Do you have a sense of how the job might evolve over time? Does it meet your professional goals? Does it put you in a good position to pursue your future professional development? Will the demands of the job work in concert with your responsibilities to your home and family? Does it feel like a "good fit"? Remember that every CNS job is unique and shaped by the facility's expectations of the role. Nonetheless, you still have major input into how the role plays out over time. Always consider the potential for how the role can be shaped and reshaped into what you want it to be.

While you are unable to read the future, you must make the decision about accepting this offer with your head, your gut, and your heart. Consider how this position meets your vision of the optimal CNS role and why you became a CNS. Review your experiences to date. Think about how those experiences, along with your passions and talents, align with the expectations of the job. Reflect upon the questions you were asked and ponder the answers to your questions during the interviews. Finally, consider how this job complements your personal life. Then, listen to your internal voice about what feels right … and decide!

REFERENCES

American Nurses Credentialing Center. (2015) *Consensus model for APRN regulation: Frequently asked questions.* Retrieved from www.nursecredentialing.org

Block, J., & Petrus, M. (2004). *Great answers! Great questions! To your job interview.* New York, NY: McGraw-Hill.

Byham, W., & Pickett, D. (1999). *Landing the job you want.* New York, NY: Three Rivers Press.

Career Consulting Corner. (n.d.). *Interview preparation Area 2.* Retrieved from http://www.careercc.com/interv3.shtml

Fitzwater, T. (2001). *Preparing for the behavior based interview.* Menlo Park, CA: Crisp Publications.

Hansens, K. (n.d.). Quintessential Careers. *Behavioral job interviewing strategies for job-seekers.* Retrieved from www.quintcareers.com/behvioral_interviewing.html

Hartigan, C. (2011). APRN regulation: The licensure-certification interface. *AACN Advanced Critical Care, 22* (1), 50–65.

Kessler, R. (2006). *Competency based interviews: Master the tough new interview style.* Franklin Lakes, NJ: Career Press.

National Council of State Boards of Nursing. (2010). *APRN consensus model: Frequently asked questions.* Retrieved from www.ncsbn.org/736.htm

Pohly, P. (n.d.). *Successfully answer behavioral questions in your job interview.* Retrieved from http://www.pohly.com/interview-3.html

Powers, L. (2000). Anatomy of an interview. *AORN, 72* (4), 671–674.

Quintessential Careers. (n.d.). *STAR interviewing response technique for success in behavioral job interviews.* Retrieved from www.quintcareers.com/STAR_interviewing

U.S. Department of Labor. (2005, December 20). *Bureau of Labor statistics occupational outlook handbook: Job interview tips.* Retrieved from http://www.bls.gov/oco/oco20045.htm

Welton, R. H., Morton, P. G., & Amig, A. (1998). How to succeed in job interviewing. *Critical Care Nurse, 18* (1), 68–73.

CHAPTER 2

Creating a Job Description

KATHLEEN M. VOLLMAN
DENISE O'BRIEN
CATHY C. LEWIS

The job description for the clinical nurse specialist (CNS) is the foundation for practice of the role within the organization where the CNS is employed. A job description needs to be general enough to be inclusive of all variations of CNS practice, but specific enough to serve as a roadmap for the essential role components to be actualized. In addition, a job description identifies the basic parameters for performance appraisal. If no job description exists, one should be created. Existing job descriptions should be reviewed and updated every several years.

Fundamentally, a job description is an outline of the essential characteristics of the CNS role and includes minimal requirements for safe practice, such as education, certification, and experience. To achieve timely development or updating of a job description, one should focus on a consensus-building process and use of evidence. The following is a list of suggested strategies to get started:

1. Use national CNS core competencies as a foundation for the development of the CNS job description (nacns.org/html/competencies.php).
2. Review the various types of CNS practice within the institution, such as unit-based, program-based, inpatient, or outpatient.
3. Create a committee that includes representation from differing types of CNS practice and nursing administration, including both frontline manager and director level administrators. Consider including a staff nurse representative.

CREATING THE JOB DESCRIPTION

Using national CNS core competencies as the foundation for the job description helps keep the job description within professional, agreed-upon boundaries. National core competencies help define the scope and practice of the CNS role regardless of specialty, and ensure that entry-level key characteristics and competencies are incorporated. Every job description should have an organizing framework. The National Association of Clinical Nurse Specialists (NACNS, 2004) created a conceptual model in which the competencies of the CNS role are described. The framework is called the "three spheres of influence." The three spheres include the patient/client sphere, the nurses/ practice sphere, and the organization/system sphere. The framework provides flexibility and recognizes that CNS practice may be actualized differently based on the CNS specialty, setting, population, and/or organizational needs. The revised national competencies (2010) continue to use the three spheres of influence as one of the organizing frameworks (nacns.org/html/competencies.php).

COMPONENTS OF THE JOB DESCRIPTION

In most health care agencies, components of a CNS or professional job description are organized by a pre-existing format from the human resources department. A job description typically consists of several major components: a general overview or summary section, principal duties and responsibilities, qualifications, required and desired skills, and abilities/ competencies (University of Pittsburgh—Office of Human Resources, n.d., Appendix 2.1).

The Position Summary

The position summary is a brief description (three to five sentences) of the overall duties and responsibilities associated with the role. Position summaries may include information about the amount of freedom or independence the role has, existing partnerships, as well as to whom the person holding the job reports (University of Pittsburgh–Office of Human Resources, n.d.). The position summary helps answer the question: Why does this job exist?

Principal Duties and Responsibilities

The principal duties and responsibilities section is the heart of the job description. It captures *what you would do* or the fundamental purpose of the job and associated duties. Performance standards or competencies describe the expectations of how the job is to be performed (University of Pittsburgh–Office of Human Resources, n.d.). Using an organizing framework, such as the three spheres of influence, helps create distinction for the various functional role competencies and job responsibilities. The words used to describe the job role and actions should be higher level verbs such as "compare and contrast," "design," "evaluate," "establish," "mentor," and "lead."

Required Qualifications

The required qualifications section should specify required educational preparation, experience, and licensure. The education qualification component can be challenging to write because of the different levels of educational preparation for CNSs that have occurred over the years. It was not until 1998, with the first publication of the *Statement on Clinical Nurse Specialist Practice and Education*, that a more definitive outline for classroom and clinical education specifically for the CNS existed (NACNS, 1998). Additional structure was added through the advanced practice registered nurse (APRN) consensus document that helped to create consistency for entry level of practice for all four advanced practice roles at the role and population levels. For recognition, many states are working to adopt the APRN consensus model that requires CNSs to be certified by a professional nursing organization in addition to holding a graduate degree. Eligibility requirements for certification often include 500 supervised clinical hours completed within an educational program. Prior to the late 1990s, most programs' clinical hour requirement was less than 500 hours, leaving some long-practicing CNSs ineligible for most certification examinations. In addition, many clinical specialty areas do not offer certification options at the advanced practice level. Addressing issues of certification in a job description requires considered thought based on what is occurring at the state and national levels. Legal requirements differ among the states as progress continues toward title recognition and scope of practice descriptions for CNSs.

The goal of a job description is to ensure that each employee meets the minimum educational requirements for safety to practice at an advanced level. Trying to achieve balance among educational preparation, legal requirements, and a sufficient number of available qualified candidates is tricky. The example job description demonstrates one method of achieving that balance in a state that does not have title protection (Appendix 2.1) but is working toward adoption of the APRN consensus model. Minimum experience as a nurse and as a CNS needs to be clearly identified. The title "CNS" denotes being an expert in a clinical specialty at an advanced level. Therefore, level of expertise in a clinical specialty and how that expertise will be achieved and maintained need to be described in the required qualifications section.

Skills and Abilities

The skills and abilities portion of the job description specifies minimum competencies required for job performance. Skills for the APRN include leadership, communication, collaboration, mentoring, and leading change. These are the essential characteristics of the CNS role outlined in the NACNS *Statement on Clinical Nurse Specialist Practice and Education* (2004), as well as part of the National CNS Core Competencies document (NACNS, 2010). Abilities are those personal characteristics an employee has that may be needed to excel in a job. A CNS should be able to demonstrate the ability to utilize evidence to develop, teach, guide, and implement practice standards and policies. These skills and abilities should be verified through a portfolio, recommendation letters, the interview process, and/or demonstration.

Desired Qualifications

The final components listed in the job description are those qualifications that are desired but not required. Desired additional qualifications can be used as a strategy to help determine the better candidate when two or more job applicants meet all the required qualifications for the job. Some examples of desired qualifications include certification in an area of clinical specialty, experience as a CNS for more than 5 years, and skills using various computer applications including databases, data mining, and information technology. Desired qualifications can often tip the scales during the hiring process if there is competition between applicants with similar required qualifications.

CONTROVERSIES AND PRACTICAL SOLUTIONS

Educational preparation, key clinical experience, and reporting structure are essential components of any CNS job description; however, these content areas may create controversy during the development phase. Defining educational preparation for a CNS can be challenging due to the historical and current variability of CNS educational programs across the country (Hamric, Hanson, Tracy, & O'Grady, 2013). CNS educational programs today should be accredited and should address national recommendations for course content and clinical experiences outlined by the American Association of Colleges of Nursing's *Essentials of Master's Education* (2011) and the NACNS's *Statement on Clinical Nurse Specialist Practice and Education* (2004), as well as the Clinical Nurse Specialist Core Competencies document (NACNS, 2010). In addition, this would include a minimum of 500 hours of supervised (by a CNS) clinical experience. The CNS applicant who has recently completed a graduate program that meets recommendations should be able to pass the appropriate CNS certification for a specific population focus and enter into CNS practice. Curricula for some population foci (e.g., pediatrics) are currently undergoing further revision for alignment with the full implementation of the APRN Consensus Model. Each organization must evaluate language to address privileging and credentialing if the CNS has prescriptive authority and the organization wishes to incorporate it within the CNS role.

Performance evaluations may be used to determine any deficits that could be resolved through continuing education or continuing clinical precepted experiences. CNS applicants should possess a minimum level of nursing practice experience and expertise in the clinical specialty area. The expectation of demonstrated clinical expertise should occur within 6 months to 1 year of hire. Without this expectation, the CNS may have difficulty fully operationalizing the CNS role of expert clinical practitioner.

In situations where there are not enough CNS candidates to fill open positions, it is important to avoid accepting candidates who do not meet the requirements in the job description or who do not have experience in the population focus. There may be limited candidates to interview for some CNS specialties in some states, which may require a national search for qualified CNSs. Conversely, any CNS being interviewed should look carefully at the job description at the prospective institution or facility to ensure that it supports the candidate's practice as a CNS. Another area of controversy includes reporting relationships. A CNS, as an advanced practice nurse, should report to a nursing administrator with an advanced degree. Variations on reporting relationships will exist, and reporting relationships are highly dependent on the organization's administrative structure. Within complex organizations, the primary need is for consistency in the reporting structure. By standardizing the reporting relationships, the CNS position is strengthened and supported throughout the organization.

Because the role of the CNS is essentially that of expert in clinical practice and support for the bedside nurse in the provision of the highest quality nursing care, the CNS should lead clinical practice for the unit, program, or area. Partnering the CNS and the nurse manager provides optimal unit or program leadership. The CNS and the nurse manager work as partners to support the clinical nursing practice of the unit or across a program. Collaboration promotes best practices and supports positive nursing outcomes. Joint meetings to identify each partner's role, discuss potential concerns, and offer models of working CNS/nurse manager partnerships also help support the CNS and the nurse manager. Clearly articulating the CNS role components for nurse managers and other leaders may help decrease resistance to these partnerships. Illustrating the potential value and outcomes of successful partnerships will educate CNSs and nurse managers unfamiliar with each other's role and will help them work together successfully in the future.

Once consensus is reached regarding any controversial areas, the job description is complete. The next step is to submit the document to administration and human resources for final approval. While that review is underway, the group can begin to look at creating the interview process, orientation, and performance appraisal.

USING THE CNS JOB DESCRIPTION TO DEVELOP OTHER CNS TOOLS

A carefully crafted CNS job description that is based on national core competencies and that reflects the needs for CNS practice in a particular organization becomes an invaluable foundation for the development of other tools related to the CNS role. The CNS core competencies and responsibilities in each of the three spheres of influence that are detailed in the job description provide a consistent structure for the CNS interview process, the CNS orientation program, and the CNS performance evaluation.

CNS Interview Process

Candidates for CNS positions should be initially screened to ensure that they meet the required qualifications for educational preparation and experience that are specified in the job description. Nursing directors can clarify whether a candidate has the appropriate graduate or doctoral degree with required CNS competencies. Those candidates who meet the required qualifications can be further evaluated though interviews, portfolio reviews, and letters of recommendation.

The interview process should have a broad base of participation from staff that will interface directly with the CNS, including the nursing director, nurse manager, staff nurses, other CNSs, and select multidisciplinary team members. Participation by multiple interviewers can be facilitated through the use of a structured interview tool with discussion items and questions based on core competencies in each of the three spheres of influence. These discussion points will help evaluate the candidate's strengths in advanced practice skills of leadership, communication, collaboration, mentoring, and change management. For example:

Direct Patient Care
- Describe skills that are necessary to work with various groups.
- Talk about a time when you used these skills in a patient care situation. (team building/collaboration, communication, leadership)

Nursing/Nursing Practice
- Give an example of a time when you used evidence or performance improvement to change nursing practice or standardize care at the institutional level. (leadership, clinical expertise, communication, problem solving, change management, mentoring)

Organization/System
- What issue do you think will have the most impact on the way nursing is practiced in the future? (professional development, leadership)

A structured recording tool should be used to allow interview participants to record impressions of the candidate's answers. A portfolio can be very helpful in demonstrating the candidate's prior experiences and skill sets in many areas of CNS practice. The candidate can also be asked to provide brief educational presentations as a part of the interview with staff nurses.

CNS Orientation Program

The CNS orientation program is based on achieving competencies that are derived directly from the responsibilities listed in the CNS job description. The structural framework is again the three spheres of CNS practice. The orientation should also incorporate adult-learning principles and be customized to meet the individual needs of the CNS orientee. At the heart of an orientation program is the guidance and mentoring by a CNS preceptor assigned to the orientee for the duration of the orientation period. Tools might include a CNS skills inventory and a competencies/resource list. The orientee could use the skills inventory to identify and prioritize areas for further development. The orientee and the CNS preceptor could use the competencies/resource list to identify aspects of the CNS role on which to focus during orientation and the corresponding resources that may be used to help the orientee achieve competency in those areas. The length of the orientation is customized according to the needs of the orientee. The orientee's achievement of the competencies is evaluated jointly by the orientee, the CNS preceptor, the nurse manager, and the nursing director. The orientee is also asked to evaluate the orientation program itself to facilitate program improvement. If the CNS has prescriptive authority, the privileging and credentialing process required for the organization should occur within the orientation time frame. See Chapter 5 for more in-depth discussion of CNS orientation.

CNS Performance Evaluation

The annual evaluation of the performance of a CNS provides an opportunity to obtain feedback from the customer base. A useful tool could be a brief CNS customer survey that allows customers to rate the CNS's performance on some of the key role responsibilities and to rank the importance of each of those functions to the customer. The CNS may use a CNS performance evaluation rating tool to self-assess performance in all three spheres of influence: direct care, nurse/nursing practice, and organization/system leadership. The ratings are divided into four categories of performance: "not met," "approaching," "solid performance," and "exemplary." Sample behaviors are described under each category to assist in the rating process. The focus of behaviors in the three spheres will fluctuate for each CNS depending on the annual goals developed in partnership with the nursing director and the nurse manager partner.

The CNS job description is the starting point for the development of all of the tools described previously. There are major advantages to this development approach. Since the job description is founded on national core competencies of CNS practice, the other tools will then be aligned with core competencies. In addition, the consistent use of the same core competencies and role responsibilities in all of these documents sets a high standard for CNS performance while allowing for individual variation to meet the demands in different practice settings. Finally, the structural framework of the three spheres of influence defines and facilitates CNS participation in the full scope of CNS practice.

REFERENCES

American Association of Colleges of Nursing. (2011). *The essentials of master's education for advanced practice nursing.* Washington, DC: Author. Retrieved from http://www.aacn.nche.edu/education-resources/MastersEssentials11.pdf

Hamric, A. B., Hanson, C. M., Tracy, M. F., & O'Grady, E. T. (2013). *Advanced practice nursing: An integrative approach* (5th ed.). St. Louis, MO: Elsevier Saunders.

National Association of Clinical Nurse Specialists (NACNS). (1998). *Statement on clinical nurse specialist practice and education* (1st ed.). Harrisburg, PA: Author.

National Association of Clinical Nurse Specialists (NACNS). (2004). *Statement on clinical nurse specialist practice and education* (2nd ed.). Harrisburg, PA: Author.

National CNS Competency Task Force. (2010). *Clinical nurse specialist core competencies: Executive summary 2006–2008*. Philadelphia, PA: NACNS.

University of Pittsburgh—Office of Human Resources. (n.d.). *Job description writing guide*. Retrieved from http://www.hr.pitt.edu/sites/default/files/documents/comp/pdf/jdHow ToWrite_printerFriendly.pdf

APPENDIX 2.1 Clinical Nurse Specialist Job Description: Position Summary/Essential Characteristics

The clinical nurse specialist (CNS) is the clinical leader for a program or area of nursing practice. The advanced knowledge and skills required for this role include clinical expertise in a focus area, evidence-based practice, collaboration, consultation, education, mentoring, and change leadership. These are essential to advance the practice of nursing and the professional development of nurses. The specialized knowledge and skills are used within three major areas of focus: patient/family, nurses and nursing practice, and the organization/system. The CNS and the nurse manager are partners in leading the nursing clinical practice area. The CNS coordinates and guides clinical activities/projects of nurses within a practice area. The CNS is accountable for collaborating with members of the health care team to design, implement, and measure safe, cost-effective, evidence-based care strategies. The CNS is responsible for maintaining current professional knowledge and competencies and contributing to the advancement of the practice of nursing at the unit/system, local, state and/or national and international levels.

Responsibilities
Direct Patient Care
1. Serves as a reliable source of information on the latest evidence supporting cost-effective, safe nursing practices.
2. Collaborates with the multidisciplinary team using the nursing process to integrate the nursing perspective into a comprehensive plan of care for the patient/family.
3. Identifies and prioritizes nursing care needs for a select population of patients/families.
4. Conducts comprehensive, holistic wellness and illness assessments using established or innovative evidence-based techniques, tools, and methods.
5. Provides pharmacological and nonpharmacological treatment strategies for individual patients or populations of patients.
6. Initiates and plans care conferences or programs for individual patients or populations of patients.
7. Designs and evaluates innovative educational programs for patients, families, and groups.

(continued)

APPENDIX 2.1 Clinical Nurse Specialist Job Description: Position Summary/Essential Characteristics (*continued*)

8. Identifies, collects, and analyzes data that serve as a basis for program design and outcome measurement.
9. Establishes methods to evaluate and document nursing interventions.
10. Evaluates the impact of nursing interventions on fiscal and human resources.

Nursing/Nursing Practice
1. Collaborates with others to resolve issues related to patient care, communication, policies, and resources.
2. Creates and revises nursing policies, protocols, and procedures using evidence-based information to achieve outcomes for indicators that are nurse sensitive.
3. Identifies facilitators and addresses barriers that affect patient outcomes.
4. Leads clinical practice and quality improvement initiatives for a unit or a program.
5. Collaborates with nurses to develop practice environments that support shared decision making.
6. Assists the staff in developing critical thinking and clinical judgment.
7. Creates a nursing care environment that stimulates continuous self-learning, reflective practice, feeling of ownership, and demonstration of responsibility and accountability.
8. Collaborates with educational nurse specialists, educational nurse coordinators, and others on content and operational design of orientation, clinical competency, and other clinical educational program development.
9. Mentors nurses to acquire new skills, develop their careers, and effectively incorporate evidence into practice.
10. Provides input for staff evaluation.
11. Provides formal and informal education for nurses and other health professionals and health professional students.
12. Leads in the conduct and utilization of nursing research.

Organization/System Leadership
1. Consults with other units and health care professionals to improve care.
2. Leads/assists institutional groups to enhance the clinical practice of nurses and improve patient outcomes.
3. Develops, pilots, evaluates, and incorporates innovative models of practice across the continuum of care.
4. Designs and evaluates programs and initiatives that are congruent with the organization's strategic plans, regulatory agency requirements, and nursing standards.
5. Participates in need identification, selection, and evaluation of products and equipment.
6. Advances nursing practice through participation in professional organizations, publications, and presentations.

(*continued*)

APPENDIX 2.1 Clinical Nurse Specialist Job Description: Position Summary/Essential Characteristics (*continued*)

Required Qualifications

Education

Graduate degree (master's or doctorate) in nursing with CNS competencies. Certification in the CNS role and population is required. Some states may require a second license.

Experience

■ Minimum of 3 years clinical nursing experience is required.
■ Clinical knowledge in specialty area. If hired in an area with a substantially different clinical knowledge set, the candidate will be expected to demonstrate clinical expertise in the practice area within a 6-month to 1-year time frame.

Skills

■ Demonstrated skills at the level of an advanced practice nurse in leadership, communication, collaboration, mentoring, and change as evidenced by the candidate's portfolio, recommendation letters, references, interview, and demonstration.
■ Demonstrated ability at the level of an advanced practice nurse to utilize evidence to develop, teach, guide, and implement practice standards and policies.

Desired Qualifications

■ Advanced practice certification as a CNS.
■ Certification in area of clinical specialty.
■ Clinical nursing experience within the past 5 years.
■ Skill using various computer applications: Microsoft Office application, data mining, and general information technology.

As defined by the National Association of Clinical Nurse Specialists (2004, pp. 42–43).

CHAPTER 3

Finding a Place in the Organization

JAN POWERS

Clinical nurse specialists (CNSs) are vital to building a health care system that is evidence-based, patient-centered, safe, ethical, outcomes-focused, and cost-effective (Heitkemper, 2004). Sometimes, finding a place in the organizational structure can be a source of frustration for the new CNS. This is especially true with the changing environment of health care organizations. The following information will assist you in your quest for a CNS position that meets your own professional needs as well as the needs of an organization to provide safe, high-quality, cost-effective care to patients.

COMPLEXITY OF HEALTH CARE SYSTEMS

The complexity of health care systems has increased dramatically in the past several decades (McKeon, 2006). The health care environment continues to evolve with health care reform and implementation of the Affordable Care Act. The intricate nature of health care in highly complex environments, both inpatient and outpatient, requires multiple team members to manage patient care, making it imperative that effective communication and interprofessional collaboration occur. The culture within an organization will determine its ability to function and produce high-quality outcomes. A strong culture facilitates high performance. A system of shared values allows employees to apply these values to benefit the organization as a whole. The foundation of a strong culture in health care is trust among disciplines, collaboration, and communication (McDougall, 1987). Communication is the process of sharing information with people that increases their understanding. Trust and collaboration involve understanding and valuing each role's unique contributions and the ability to work together to attain the best outcomes for patient care (McDougall, 1987).

Interdisciplinary collaboration is essential in health care settings. Lack of communication and collaboration has been shown to be responsible for as much as 70% of the adverse events currently reported (Fewster-Thuente & Velsor-Friedrich, 2008). Some elements that are essential for successful inter-disciplinary collaboration are interprofessional education, role awareness, and interpersonal relationship skills (Petri, 2010). Therefore, in order to facilitate communication and collaboration, it is essential that all team members under-stand the responsibilities of each other's roles so that they can effectively work together.

DIFFERENT DISCIPLINES AND ROLES

Each different discipline has its own knowledge base, behaviors, and standards of practice (Orchard, 2005). Each member of the team brings a different set of values, personal experiences, and beliefs. In order to develop trust for collaborative practice to occur, role clarification and role valuing are required (McKeon, 2006).

Roles need to be clearly delineated through job descriptions that provide the expectations of each position. If roles are not clearly defined, role conflict may occur. Role conflict and role ambiguity create stress and diminish the effectiveness of the organization (McDougall, 1987). In a highly effective organization, all professionals are valued and recognized as possess-ing the intellectual and moral capital necessary to provide excellent patient care (McKeon, 2006).

The CNS is an integral part of an organization and brings a unique clinical focus to his or her practice. The CNS role historically involves many differ-ent role components, including leader, educator, researcher, and consultant. Because of these many different aspects, the CNS role may be confused with other roles within an organization. It is imperative that a new CNS understands other roles in the organization and clearly delineates and explains to others the unique qualities of the CNS role.

The CNS role may overlap with other disciplines, such as educators, case managers, quality liaisons, clinical managers, and clinical pharmacists. The role and goals of the CNS's practice must be clearly identified and defined for other disciplines to understand. Therefore, it is imperative for the new CNS to not only articulate his or her role and responsibilities, but to understand other roles within the institution and how to integrate his or her position into the institution. Variation of roles may exist among different institutions, so it is important to ascertain job functions and duties and to be able to verbalize how the CNS can collaborate with each specific discipline.

Nurse Educator

The CNS role is often confused with the educator role; in fact, some institutions have attempted to combine the educator and CNS roles into one job category. This typically has not worked well and should be discouraged because the role of educator usually becomes the primary focus at the expense of the clinical expert aspects of the CNS role. A nurse educator is typically focused entirely on educating and training nurses and nursing staff. Nurse educators are responsible for designing, implementing, and evaluating educational programs for nurses to prepare them to care for patients in the health care environment (Nurses for a Healthier Tomorrow, Career Info, 2015).

Case Manager

Case management is a collaborative process that assesses, plans, implements, coordinates, monitors, and evaluates options and services to meet an individual's health care needs through communication and effective resource coordination to promote quality, cost-effective outcomes across the continuum of care (American Case Management Association, 2015). Case managers may have different titles or positions depending on the institution, such as "care manager," "outcomes manager," or "care coordinator." This person guides patients through the complex health care process, providing responses to questions and connecting the patient and family to needed resources.

Quality Managers

Quality managers or liaisons use a comprehensive body of knowledge and are experts at quality agency regulations and data required to meet these mandated standards of practice. These experts in performance improvement and quality assurance should help guide and direct processes that promote safe, high-quality, cost-effective patient care (Healthcare Quality Certification Board, n.d.). The quality liaison also provides internal measurement of quality indicators and provides benchmarking for both internal and external quality indicators.

Nurse Practitioner

The nurse practitioner (NP) conducts physical examinations, orders and interprets laboratory results, selects plans of treatment, identifies medication requirements, and performs certain medical management activities for selected health conditions, usually with a focus on meeting primary health care needs (American Academy of Nurse Practitioners, 2015).

These are just a few examples of roles that may be present in any organization where a CNS may also be employed. Variations of roles exist within different organizations; therefore, it is important to ascertain role functions and duties and to be able to articulate how the CNS is differentiated from, yet can collaborate with, each specific role. The CNS can then focus on effective collaboration with all disciplines at the patient, nurse, and system levels to optimize clinical outcomes (McClelland, McCoy, & Burson, 2013).

CNS ROLE WITHIN AN ORGANIZATION

The essence of CNS practice is clinical expertise in a specialty area and in nursing practice in the care of patients with complex needs (National Association of Clinical Nurse Specialists [NACNS], 2004). CNS education includes content on role competencies within the spheres of influence (patient/client, nursing practice/nurses, system/organization). The CNS impacts patient outcomes directly through practice and indirectly through the influence of nursing practice at the bedside. The CNS assists staff in impacting practice by creating an environment that promotes the empowerment of nursing (DeBourgh, 2001). The CNS role-models advanced nursing practice by interacting confidently with physicians, demonstrating flexibility in complex situations, incorporating the feedback of others before reaching a decision, and demonstrating accountability (DeBourgh, 2001).

Through evidence-based nursing care standards and programs of care, a CNS influences nurses (NACNS, 2004). He or she can also influence systems to mobilize, change, or transform in order to facilitate expertly designed nursing interventions targeted toward achieving quality, cost-effective, patient-focused outcomes (NACNS, 2004). The application of the nursing process at an advanced practice level and execution of clinical decision making are integral to the role of the CNS. The CNS develops innovative solutions while acting as a change agent, assists nursing staff with decision making in clinical situations, and promotes evidence-based clinical practice and research to optimize clinical practice.

The CNS is a champion for evidence-based practice, clinical inquiry, and nursing research that aim to improve patient outcomes specifically related to nursing practice. The CNS disseminates current research-based literature and theories necessary for the advancement of patient care. The CNS also conducts cost–benefit analyses and promotes cost-effectiveness of interventions, process improvements, and product utilization, to ensure desired outcomes and cost containment. The CNS contributes to the development of interdisciplinary standards of practice, guidelines of care, and system-level policy. Utilizing evidence-based practice and resources, CNSs develop key tools and processes that support achievement of quality outcomes for specific populations and create innovative alternative solutions to system problems.

The CNS serves as a mentor and role model for the staff. The CNS must be proficient in interpersonal skills related to communication, collaboration, change management, group process, conflict management, implementation science, and negotiation.

INTEGRATION INTO AN ORGANIZATION

The CNS may enter into a job as the only CNS in the system. If there is more than one CNS in the system, it is typical that each CNS has a different area of specialization. When a CNS enters an organization, he or she becomes a member of multiple groups within the system, including the nursing leadership team, specialty unit staff, CNS peer group, medical staff, and various multidisciplinary teams such as the coronary care team, oncology team, or rehabilitation team. Successful organizational entry depends on the new CNS making a smooth transition. This transition can be challenging as the new CNS needs to develop an understanding of the organization, including the culture, values, and history, as well as the personalities of dominant leaders (formal and informal) within the organization.

Some measured steps can be taken to ease the transition from newcomer to insider. To become an insider, a CNS must begin to recognize system norms and organizational behavior patterns, accept organizational reality, achieve role clarity, and locate oneself within the organizational context (Krcmar, 1991). Understanding organizational culture, values, and norms does not mean that a CNS must conform to the practices. It is easier to transition to an organization that holds the same values and beliefs; however, personal and organizational values do not need to totally coincide. Often a CNS may be hired to assist in changing the culture and values of an organization. If this is the case, the CNS must be an expert in the change process and must be very strong in his or her values—this may not be an optimal climate for a new CNS.

Entry into a system is a process that may take considerable time and energy. The process must be planned and deliberate with a designated time frame (Krcmar, 1991). Issues regarding role establishment and role clarification begin to emerge as a CNS enters an organization. Therefore, it is important to understand organizational structure and roles. The new CNS will undoubtedly encounter differing role expectations, and others will place varying degrees of importance on those expectations (Krcmar, 1991).

Even while mastering the CNS role components, challenges often occur for a new CNS when entering into a position where other advanced roles or other disciplines may have overlapping areas of responsibility or areas of support. The new CNS may experience role conflict and therefore struggle between being what he or she wants to be and conforming to the views others hold of the role (Krcmar, 1991). A new CNS will need to determine expectations and be able to articulate the CNS role in order to provide and reinforce clarity. This is also true if the nurse has been in an organization in a different capacity before taking a CNS position, such as moving from staff nurse to CNS. In this situation, a new CNS must establish himself or herself in a different role within existing relationships, as others may tend to view the CNS in his or her previous capacity. Reestablishing a new role in the organization will require multiple reminders and reinforcement by the new CNS.

COLLABORATION

Complex organizations require many different roles and multiple team members to effectively manage patient care. With multiple team members, it is imperative that organizations require interprofessional collaboration.

A new CNS must establish those collaborative relationships with nurses and other providers in order to establish goals and to implement a plan of care. Collaboration may be hampered by differences in professional perspectives that exist across health providers (McKeon, 2006). Successful collaboration includes mutual trust and respect, and understanding and support of each other's roles and responsibilities. Collaboration should involve a shared vision, a shared responsibility for outcomes, joint decision making, teamwork interdependency, and open communication skills (Culver-Clark & Greenawald, 2013).

A CNS in collaborative practice fosters mutual support and networking through commitments to professional interdisciplinary processes within the organization. The CNS should be focused on establishing collaborative relationships within and across departments that promote patient safety and clinical excellence.

Collaboration among all disciplines is extremely important. The most effective outcomes are developed through a collaborative approach. A CNS needs to participate with the nurse manager to plan for and implement goals related to nursing practice. He or she should assist with identifying educational needs and collaborating with nurse educators to develop targeted plans for education of nursing staff. The CNS also needs to develop mutually respected CNS–physician relationships.

A CNS may need to help physicians understand the CNS role. Physicians often relate better to the elements of an advanced practice role that is consistent with the medical model. The CNS role is often difficult for the physician to understand because of nursing's specialized focus versus medical practice. CNSs emphasize autonomous nursing practice and focus on nurse-sensitive outcomes.

A collegial relationship is built on shared knowledge, confidence, and mutual trust. An effective, well-functioning team has trust among team members, openly communicates, has shared expectations and defined roles and responsibilities, creates a shared vision, promotes disagreement while containing conflict, and uses individual strengths, talents, and values on behalf of the patient and family (Bennett & Gadlin, 2012; King, 1990).

REPORTING RELATIONSHIPS

Placement of a CNS in the organizational structure is an important consideration for a new CNS. The CNS typically does not have line authority (management authority), so he or she needs to earn the trust and respect of others to be effective. Since the CNS usually promotes change by virtue of expertise and influence rather than authority, communication skills are crucial.

Variability exists in reporting relationships of CNSs. A study by Darmody (2011) reported that much variation exists in reporting relationships for CNSs from one administrator supervising and evaluating all CNSs in a system to multiple directors supervising CNSs within their service areas.

The CNS reporting structure ideally should be outside of the unit or specialty area. If the CNS reports to a director or manager of a service area, this implies that the CNS "belongs to" that individual and may be used to meet the director's own agenda rather than being encouraged to meet the CNS's identified clinical needs. Optimally the CNS should report to a chief nursing officer or a CNS manager who is also a CNS. This type of reporting structure will enable the new CNS to gain the mentoring needed and develop a collaborative partnership with the manager or director of the unit or area for which he or she is responsible. Regardless of the reporting relationship, nursing administration support is crucial to the CNS's success.

Attention should also be given to social networks that promote information flow and influence processes in complex organizations. This has significant implications for the CNS whose role is focused on influence with patients, nurses, and organization levels (Darmody, 2011).

KEYS TO EFFECTIVE INTEGRATION

Health care environments are highly complex and changing rapidly. The ability to be innovative and work collaboratively is essential for the CNS. The CNS must understand the system/organization and be innovative and creative in order to adapt to changing health care environments (McClelland et al., 2013). CNSs play a key role in the emerging health care system. They need to demonstrate leadership on teams, and use their skill set in order to redesign the health system in a cost-effective, patient-centered approach, making it an efficient model to improving health care outcomes (McClelland et al., 2013).

Advanced practice nurses can make a complex health care environment into a solution-oriented facility rather than a blame-focused facility (Richmond, 2005). It is imperative that a CNS be able to maintain tranquility when surrounded by chaos. A CNS can affect decision making by becoming a member of strategic committees. Effective participation in patient rounds is the most direct method of influencing patient care; it is important to use patient rounds to their maximum benefit.

Even while mastering CNS practice competencies, challenges often occur for the new CNS when entering into a position. The CNS may need to determine expectations and articulate the role of the CNS to provide role clarity.

For the CNS, changing roles within an organization or changing organizations can be a stressful time. However, this can and should be a very exciting and rewarding experience for everyone involved. There are many steps that the CNS can take to ease his or her integration into the new role and/or new system; these are presented in Table 3.1. Following these key steps will afford a successful entry into an organizational structure.

These key steps will help ease the transition when the CNS enters an institution. These steps include meeting with nursing leadership, medical directors,

---

TABLE 3.1 Tips for Successful Integration of a New CNS Into a Health Care Organization

- Ensure that quality and safety are addressed with patient care and outcomes.
- Ensure reporting structures are supportive and allow for independent, innovative, and creative practice.
- Take time to understand others' roles in the organization and to build trusting relationships.
- Develop lines of communication with formal and informal leaders in the organization.
- Determine the expectations of others and find ways to collaborate with other disciplines, providers, and staff.
- Value the norms and behavior patterns of the organization.
- Align with selected individuals within the organization to create peer groups.
- Be able to articulate the CNS role, practice, and core competencies.
- Look for opportunities, such as at staff meetings, to explain the CNS role.

CNS, clinical nurse specialist.

---

educators, and other key individuals. These meetings are a forum for the CNS to introduce himself or herself, explain his or her role, and lay the foundation for collaborative practice. A CNS should spend time working with units and groups related to the specialty in order to understand current practice and to build relationships. A CNS can also hold journal clubs, attend unit meetings, and offer fliers and brochures to help others understand the role of the CNS. A new CNS needs to take the time to establish relationships and build trust, which will lay the foundation for future initiatives.

Confidence in one's role is an important contributor to success. Gaining and sharing confidence is also enhanced by establishing relationships with professional colleagues outside the workplace—professional growth is essential. Being a lifelong learner and developing relationships with peers who share strategies that work in their own organizations allow a CNS a variety of avenues to expand his or her influence.

REFERENCES

American Academy of Nurse Practitioners. (2015). *FAQ about nurse practitioners*. Retrieved from http://www.aanp.org

American Case Management Association. (2015). Retrieved from http://www.acmaweb.org/net/newsroom_links.aspx

Bennett, L. M., & Gadlin, H. (2012). Collaboration and team science: From theory to practice. *Journal of Investigative Medicine, 60*(5), 768–775.

Culver-Clark, R., & Greenawald, M. (2013). Nurse–physician leadership: Insights into interprofessional collaboration. *Journal of Nursing Adminstration, 43*(12), 653–659.

Darmody, J. V. (2011). Reporting relationships of clinical nurse. *Clinical Nurse Specialist, 25*(5), 244–252.

DeBourgh, G. (2001). Champions for evidence-based practice: A critical role for advanced practice nurses. *AACN Clinical Issues, 12* (4), 491–508.

Fewster-Thuente, L., & Velsor-Friedrich, B. (2008). Interdisciplinary collaboration for health-care professionals. *Nursing Administration Quarterly, 32*(1), 40–48.

Healthcare Quality Certification Board. (n.d.). *Certified Professional in Healthcare Quality (CPHQ) program.* Retrieved from http://www.cphq.org

Heitkemper, M. (2004). Clinical nurse specialists: State of the profession and challenges ahead. *Clinical Nurse Specialist, 18*(3), 135–140.

King, M. (1990). Clinical nurse specialist collaboration with physicians. *Clinical Nurse Specialist, 4*(4), 172–177.

Krcmar, C. (1991). Organizational entry: The case of the clinical nurse specialist. *Clinical Nurse Specialist, 5*(1), 38–42.

McClelland, M., McCoy, M. A., & Burson, R. (2013). Clinical nurse specialists then, now, and the future of the profession. *Clinical Nurse Specialist, 27*(2), 96–102.

McDougall, G. (1987). The role of the clinical nurse specialist consultant in organizational development. *Clinical Nurse Specialist, 1* (3), 133–139.

McKeon, L. O. (2006). Safeguarding patients, complexity science, high reliability organizations, and implications for team training in healthcare. *Clinical Nurse Specialist, 20*(6), 298–304.

National Association of Clinical Nurse Specialists (NACNS). (2004). *Statement on clinical nurse specialist practice and education* (2nd ed.). Harrisburg, PA: Author.

Nurses for a Healthier Tomorrow, Career Info. (2015). *Nurse Educator.* Retrieved from http://www.nursesource.org/nurse_educator.html

Orchard, C. C. (2005). Creating a culture for interdisciplinary collaborative professional practice. *Medical Education Online, 10*(11), 1–13.

Petri, L. (2010). Concept analysis of interdisciplinary collaboration. *Nursing Forum, 45,* 73–82.

Richmond, T. (2005). Creating an advanced practice nurse-friendly culture. *AACN Clinical Issues, 16*(1), 58–66.

CHAPTER 4

Working With "The Boss"

ANN M. HERBAGE BUSCH

MANAGING UP

The boss? What boss?! A motivated, independent, knowledgeable clinical nurse specialist (CNS) might want to relegate dealing with a boss to a lower priority than dealing with the day-to-day patient issues. The patient does come first; however, in order to improve patient outcomes, dealing with the boss must also be high priority, especially for the novice CNS and the CNS in a new setting. What if the boss believes that the CNS should be added into RN staffing when staffing is short ... and this happens 4 out of 5 days? Obviously, this CNS needs to deal with the boss or the CNS's goals will not get accomplished. The boss might have different ideas as to how to achieve improved patient outcomes, might prioritize differently, or might even have a different vision of the CNS job description and function than the CNS does. In addition, the boss has knowledge of economic pressures that will impact patient care and CNS role enactment. Therefore, dealing with the boss should be of utmost priority and has mutual benefits (McNichol, 2013; Scott, 2007). Some call this "managing up" (Matuson, 2011). Managing your boss may initially sound a bit manipulative or Machiavellian; however, to be an effective employee and CNS, dealing with the boss is an important and legitimate reality. Matuson (2011) believes that one's success in an organization is dependent on how well one manages the relationship with the boss.

Whether the boss is a nurse, a physician, a non-nurse and nonphysician health care administrator, or an administrator without a health care background, there are certain fundamental practices the CNS should implement in order to maximize the CNS role, not only to survive but thrive. This chapter covers the fundamentals that not only will help in dealing with the boss but will assist in successful role implementation and career achievement. Of note, there is very little written in nursing literature regarding working with the boss, and most was written more than 5 years previously. This is in alignment with the general management literature for which there is little new information. Research in this area is needed.

Many bosses draw a fine line between success and failure (Freedman, 2007). For example, at a CNS's annual performance review, instead of remembering that the CNS was successful in facilitating a dramatic decrease in surgical site infections, the boss remembers that the CNS did not develop a patient diabetic educational booklet that the boss had as a priority. The boss then marks a satisfactory score for overall performance compared to the CNS's outstanding self-rating. To avoid this negative scenario, the CNS and the boss should initially discuss the CNS's goals during orientation. Hamric and Spross (1989) believe that the heart of the relationship between the CNS and the administrator may be goal setting together. By identifying problems and establishing and prioritizing goals, the CNS and the boss expose the common purpose that binds them together, and they can plan mutual activities to attain the goals. Goals should include items for the enhancement of the CNS's individual performance as well as department and organizational goals. Goal setting for 6 months with reasonable time frames may be more useful than for 12 months in the rapidly changing health care environment (Hamric & Spross, 1989). The goals should be written, measurable, and reviewed at least monthly with the boss to track progress, note accomplishments, and revise as necessary (Tulgan, 2010). In addition, goals should be shared with others in the organization who interface with the CNS to facilitate appropriate expectations of the CNS. This latter strategy may prevent future misunderstandings regarding the CNS's role and priorities.

Misunderstandings can also be averted through supportive supervisors who understand the organizational structure and serve as advocates for the CNS. The boss can effectively introduce the CNS to the organization and key players (Hamric, Spross, & Hanson, 2005). Support from the boss is one of the strongest predictors of nurse job satisfaction (Scott, 2007). The boss is ideally someone who has credibility within the organization, is seen as a leader, works collaboratively with all departments, has influence over organizational resources, and has a different sphere of influence than the CNS (Hamric & Spross, 1989; Pearce, 2007). The boss should also have expertise in management as well as nursing care issues and have a graduate level of education. If possible, having worked with CNSs previously and having a firm understanding of the CNS role and its value would add to the success of the boss. It would also be a plus if the boss walked on water—seriously, for a strong boss–CNS partnership, the individual would most likely have a nursing background with direct care and leadership experience. The boss could be a unit nurse manager or a vice president or director of nursing. However, if the former, potential conflicts could arise in that the CNS has the scope of the organization, not just the one unit, and must be allowed flexibility to accomplish goals that are outside the unit when appropriate. Conflicts may also arise if the boss is a busy vice president or director of nursing; this level of supervisor may be too busy with hospital administrative matters to give much supervision to the CNS. Finally, the boss might be a physician, a non-nurse and nonphysician health care administrator, or an administrator without a health care background. If one of these situations is the case, it is imperative that the CNS be very clear about CNS and nursing roles so as not to become a "scut" worker, assistant to a physician, or jack of all trades. Although physicians have worked with nurses since medical school, there is often still a misunderstanding regarding the essence of nursing. By meeting regularly with the physician or other non-nurse boss to review role implementation, the CNS should be able to stay on track (Hamric & Spross, 1989; Sparacino, Cooper, & Minarik, 1990). In addition, the CNS may find it helpful to "perception check" with CNS peers (McNichol, 2013).

MORE THAN ONE BOSS

What if the CNS has more than one boss? There may be a "direct-line" boss and a "dotted line" to a boss with indirect responsibility. This often occurs when the primary boss is a non-nurse. In this instance, the CNS needs to be very aware of organizational politics and be very clear as to which boss has primary authority. Responsibility and accountability should be clearly delineated (Hamric & Spross, 1989). The primary boss has final approval of the CNS's goals, but input and approval should also be sought from the indirect boss.

TYPES OF SUPERVISION

The frequency of CNS and boss meetings and the amount of boss support the CNS requires vary with the qualities, experience, and education of the CNS. Most CNSs are committed professionals who are motivated to obtain personal success within the organization and who set difficult but achievable goals (Hamric & Spross, 1989). These qualities encourage supportive supervision, which gives the CNS freedom to determine many aspects of the role. However, supportive supervision does not mean that the CNS can do whatever he or she wants without regard to the organizational needs. With prospective communication and mutually agreed upon goals with the boss, this type of supervision allows a great deal of CNS autonomy in enacting the role with accompanying high CNS job satisfaction while still achieving organizational goals (Hamric & Spross, 1989). Despite there being a collegial and collaborative relationship between the CNS and the boss, the hierarchical chain of responsibility common to most health care organizations remains in place; the boss has administrative authority over job descriptions, operations, and evaluations (Hamric et al., 2005; Scott, 2007). For those CNSs with a lower level of maturity, less experience, or less commitment than the CNS described thus far, supervision can be increased to be more advisory and directive. This differential supervision takes the professional and role developmental level of the CNS into consideration. If this is the supervisory style used, the boss should make explicit how the CNS can achieve greater autonomy in the future (Hamric & Spross, 1989).

How often should the supervisor have scheduled meetings with the CNS? New CNSs and CNSs new to the organization usually find it beneficial to meet with the boss for 1 hour weekly to clarify expectations, discuss progress, and seek guidance (Hamric & Spross, 1989; Tulgan, 2010). Initially, the boss should be very specific and probe into the details of matters. Questions regarding strategies used, frustrations, areas of resistance, and organizational implications should be asked. Written goals, objectives, and explicit timelines should be reviewed in detail. Once the CNS demonstrates that problems are appropriately identified and prioritized, and goals, plans, intervention, and evaluation are expertly executed using excellent interpersonal skills and organizational finesse, the boss does not need to review future proposals in such detail (Hamric & Spross, 1989). In addition, frequency of meetings can be decreased. However, whether novice or experienced, all CNSs should still meet with their bosses periodically to receive ongoing feedback about clinical and leadership performance. Ongoing feedback makes explicit what the boss is thinking in terms of CNS performance and should encourage the CNS to make changes where needed. The CNS should also seek ongoing feedback from peers and should convey their valid information to the boss. Therefore, when the CNS's annual performance evaluation occurs, the CNS should not be hit with any surprises.

One significant point should be made regarding the CNS requesting meetings with the boss: Be cognizant of the boss's perception of these meetings. The boss may view an increase in frequency of meetings as a sign that the CNS is weak and needy (Freedman, 2007). To avoid these perceptions, the CNS should have a legitimate reason to meet, have a written agenda, make pertinent points concisely, omit whining, offer solutions, and conclude the meeting as quickly as possible.

FUNDAMENTAL PRACTICES FOR EFFECTIVELY WORKING WITH THE BOSS

Meetings with the boss can be stressful and even painful if a pleasant, healthy working relationship has not been established between the CNS and the boss. This relationship is one of the most important working relationships the CNS will have and deserves attention (Freedman, 2007; Matuson, 2011). To establish an amiable relationship, "manage up" effectively, and be a great employee, the CNS should follow nine fundamental practices for effectively working with the boss (Bruzzese, 2007; Freedman, 2007; Matuson, 2011, Pearce, 2007; Scott, 2007) (see Table 4.1).

TABLE 4.1 Fundamental Practices for the CNS Working With the Boss

1. Know the organization and the boss.
2. Make a great first impression and a lasting stellar reputation.
3. Be an excellent communicator.
4. Manage one's self.
5. Build good rapport with the boss.
6. Understand and use the attributes that the boss has to offer.
7. Offer CNS attributes to the boss.
8. Treat the boss fairly.
9. Give the boss support, compliments, and appreciation.

CNS, clinical nurse specialist.

First, the CNS needs to get to know the organization and the boss (Pearce, 2007; Scott, 2007). Some topics to consider investigating are: Is the organization for-profit or not-for-profit? Is it part of a larger multiorganizational structure? What are the patient demographics? What specialties are offered? What is the organizational culture? How does the CNS position fit into the organization? Are there other CNSs and a CNS peer group? Where does the boss fit into the organization? What are the boss's current goals, priorities, resources, and constraints? Is the boss laid back or hyperactive? Is afternoon the boss's most productive and approachable time of day? The CNS should try to better understand the boss in terms of role and personality. The CNS should observe, listen, and ask questions of other employees as well as take some time to talk with the boss about the boss's background with the organization and career goals. By learning more about the boss's world, the CNS gains insight into what the boss needs from the CNS and what might be expected. The CNS also gains insight into how to optimally interact with the boss. For instance, if mornings are not the best time of day for the boss, the CNS should not make an 8 a.m. appointment to discuss a controversial idea.

Second, the CNS needs to make a great first impression and then follow it up by building a lasting stellar reputation (Freedman, 2007). From the first interaction, impressions are made. The first impression might not even start with an in-person interaction but with an e-mail to a recruiter before the CNS is interviewed. Impressions often take into account dress, general grooming and appearance, language used, body language, and more (Freedman, 2007). Seemingly inconsequential things such as a weak handshake can give a negative first impression. According to a 1971 study by Dr. Albert Mehrabian, a pioneer in the field of verbal and nonverbal communication, people are influenced less by what another says than by how the person says it; 93% of a person's impact comes from things other than the actual words (Freedman, 2007). The CNS should be mindful of the first impression he or she is making and ensure that it reinforces what the CNS bills himself or herself to be. After this initial impression is formed, a series of further impressions is created over the next 6 months that coalesce into a reputation (Freedman, 2007). Once the reputation is formed, it is difficult to change, so the first 6 months of employment are especially critical. Creating a reputation can be seen as an opportunity for the new CNS. By consistently demonstrating the characteristics of integrity, dependability, trustworthiness, approachability, motivation, being clinically expert, good at problem solving, and showing a positive attitude, the CNS will develop a reputation as a stellar integral member of the organization. Although building this reputation might sound somewhat formidable, it is built one day at a time. Once the reputation is formed, the CNS cannot slack off or become unapproachable, because over time, the reputation can change.

The third fundamental of being a great employee and managing up is to be an excellent communicator. Possibly foremost, this means being a good listener. Because the average rate of speaking is 125 to 150 words a minute, and listening comprehension is approximately 400 to 500 words a minute, there is a listening gap where the mind can wander (Bruzzese, 2007). Therefore, the CNS must make a conscious decision to listen intently and focus totally on the words and speaker. Making good eye contact with the speaker, smiling when appropriate, and summarizing what was just heard usually indicate a good listener (Bruzzese, 2007; Freedman, 2007). In addition, a good listener is comfortable with silence; when a CNS asks a question, the CNS allows the boss to consider it and respond (McNichol, 2013). On the other hand, a poor listener often interrupts others. Interrupting implies that what the interrupter has to say is more important and is not truly listening (Bruzzese, 2007; Freedman, 2007). If the interruption is to finish the speaker's sentences, even if it is to give support to what the speaker is saying, such as, "I know how you feel," it is considered rude and changes the focus from the speaker to the interrupter. Another indication of being a poor listener is fidgeting or doodling when someone else is talking. These activities indicate that the listener is not totally focused on the speaker and is distracted (Bruzzese, 2007).

Besides being a good listener, the good communicator does not ramble or dominate the conversation. Rambling may indicate nervousness, immaturity, insecurity, or a need to be the center of attention (Freedman, 2007), attributes not associated with an effective CNS. A good communicator is aware that e-mails must be treated with respect: Never put anything in writing that should not be seen by the boss or anyone else in the organization. Because each individual has a favored form of communicating, the CNS should discuss with the boss and then employ the style of communication the boss prefers (McNichol, 2013; Tulgan, 2010). Is it e-mail, memos, sound bites, or long face-to-face discussions? If it is a written form of communication, the CNS must ensure that words are spelled correctly and proper grammar is used; if not, the CNS looks sloppy (Bruzzese, 2007; Freedman, 2007). By communicating effectively with the boss, the CNS facilitates a healthy working relationship and positively impacts his or her performance appraisal and career (Scott, 2007).

The fourth fundamental for effectively working with the boss is for the CNS to manage himself or herself and be the kind of employee bosses love (Freedman, 2007; Tulgan, 2010). This encompasses a multitude of elements, from time to technology to attitude. One way the CNS manages self is by doing his or her job well. The CNS must perform the job that the boss wants the CNS to do, not necessarily what the CNS thinks he or she should do (Matuson, 2011; McNichol, 2013; Tulgan, 2010). Establishing measurable goals together is the key to managing this potential dilemma. The CNS needs to meet all deadlines, keep his or her word, have good follow-through, and be a trusted and loyal ally. Time must be productively managed so that priorities are completed—there are only so many hours in a day, and the CNS often has more on his or her plate than is possible to accomplish. Also in managing self, the CNS needs to be prepared for all meetings, especially those with the boss. The CNS should arrive to meetings on time, have all necessary facts and details available, and present in an orderly objective fashion (Matuson, 2011; Pearce, 2007). Technology such as cell phones and e-mails needs to be managed; the CNS must establish rules with family and friends as to when to call or when messages can be returned. Personal e-mails should not be dealt with during business hours (Bruzzese, 2007). Finally, when managing one's self, an enthusiastic and positive attitude is one of the most important elements that bosses look for (Freedman, 2007; Matuson, 2011). The CNS with a positive attitude demonstrates it by starting work on time, working hard and showing that he or she cares about the job, not getting defensive when constructive criticism is offered, not gossiping, using a sense of humor, and not blaming others when things do not work out as expected (Bruzzese, 2007; Freedman, 2007; Matuson, 2011). The bottom line for fulfilling the fourth fundamental practice is that the CNS manages self so well that the boss's job is easier: Multiple demands are not made on the boss's time to manage the CNS.

Fundamental practice number five entails having the CNS build a good rapport with the boss. Since the relationship with the boss is one of the most essential components to nursing job satisfaction, this deserves attention and time to develop. Having regularly scheduled meetings with the boss provides time and a forum to better understand each other, establish a bond, and thereby work more effectively together. Scott (2007) suggests viewing the boss as a client or patient since nurses extend themselves to meet their patients' or clients' needs and should be doing the same for the boss. Showing respect for the boss will encourage the boss to respect the CNS (Pearce, 2007). Sometimes people do not bond right away. If this is the case with the CNS and the boss, the CNS should persist in trying to develop rapport and remember that developing strong relationships with friends takes months and sometimes years (Freedman, 2007).

The sixth fundamental practice for the CNS to effectively work with the boss is to understand and use what the boss has to offer (Matuson, 2011; Pearce, 2007). The boss will have attributes and organizational power that the CNS may not have. For instance, the boss might have easier access to power and influence, more experience, greater status, more control over resources, a broader vision of the organization, and greater knowledge of the politics and inner workings of the organization. When working on developing and achieving goals, the CNS should tap into these areas as appropriate. For instance, the boss should be accountable for facilitating a proper orientation and successful integration into the organization, arranging for an office and other essential items such as a phone and a computer, providing another viewpoint on issues or guidance in dealing with a difficult situation, and providing active support on projects. The boss should also be expected to provide clear expectations of the CNS role, give ongoing feedback regarding the CNS's performance, and complete the CNS's annual performance appraisal.

Just as the boss has attributes to offer the CNS, the CNS has attributes to offer the boss (Matuson, 2011; Pearce, 2007). This is fundamental number seven for effectively working with the boss. Some CNS attributes include clinical expertise, a greater and more detailed understanding of the day-to-day issues relating to the team and patients, more up-to-date knowledge regarding clinical issues, and a more informal relationship with nurses and other health care team members. The CNS should keep the boss informed of developments in his or her work so that the boss does not hear of them from others; the boss wants to hear it from the source and not be surprised. In addition, by keeping the boss informed, the CNS demonstrates a strong sense of responsibility and the ability to communicate clearly. The CNS should also offer to be the link to interpret economic realities and administrative decisions to staff nurses and clinical realities to administrators (Hamric & Spross, 1989). Anything the CNS can do to make the boss's job easier will be valued by the boss (Freedman, 2007). By offering to contribute and work hard for the team as well as by acknowledging appreciation for any opportunity to learn from the boss, the CNS sets this fundamental practice into action.

The eighth fundamental practice for the CNS is to treat the boss fairly: Do not criticize or complain about the boss and do not go over the boss's head (Matuson, 2011; McNichol, 2013; Pearce, 2007). Despite choosing a "safe" person in whom to vent frustrations or complaints about the boss, this information seems to eventually get back to the boss. The boss then loses trust in the CNS, which undermines the whole working relationship. If the CNS has an issue with the boss, the issue should be openly discussed with the boss in a scheduled meeting and suggestions for resolution given. While criticism of the boss can break the working relationship, so can going over the boss's head. In the business world, the hierarchical chain of command should be respected and protocol should be followed when communicating; otherwise the CNS alienates himself or herself from the boss and potentially from the boss's colleagues (Tulgan, 2010). The CNS should go over the boss's head only in very serious circumstances such as harassment. If this type of situation occurs, the CNS should first seek guidance from the human resources department.

The ninth and final fundamental practice in dealing with the boss is that the boss needs support, compliments, and appreciation just as the CNS does (Bruzzese, 2007; Pearce, 2007). Support can be given in ways such as assisting the boss with any priority project, telling others about the boss's strengths, and functioning as an exemplary CNS in the organization. Compliments should be sincere, specific, and not manipulative. Legitimate appreciation can put a smile on the boss and brighten everyone's day.

Following these nine fundamental practices may not be enough to guide the CNS to successful dealings with the boss if the boss has a personality that is truly toxic (Tulgan, 2010). If the boss is more than difficult, the CNS can fall into common but unhelpful coping methods such as avoiding interaction, calling in sick, or quitting the job (Scott, 2007). Instead of coping in these ways, the CNS should read resources that address specific toxic behaviors such as in Tulgan's book (2010), and implement suggested strategies. If this approach does not help the situation, the CNS is advised to seek advice from a professional in the human resource department (Scott, 2007; Tulgan, 2010).

SUMMARY

Dealing with the boss may initially seem to take time away from dealing with important patient issues. However, dealing with the boss is a crucial and legitimate concern, which will actually facilitate and provide more time for improving patient outcomes in the long run. By "managing up" effectively, the CNS can maximize CNS role implementation. In addition, the CNS and the boss can develop a successful, strong, and mutually beneficial relationship.

REFERENCES

Bruzzese, A. (2007). *Forty-five things you do that drive your boss crazy … and how to avoid them.* New York, NY: Penguin Group.

Freedman, E. (2007). *Work 101: Learning the ropes of the workplace without hanging yourself.* New York, NY: Bantam Dell.

Hamric, A. B., & Spross, J. A. (1989). *The clinical nurse specialist in theory and practice* (2nd ed.). Philadelphia, PA: W. B. Saunders.

Hamric, A. B., Spross, J. A., & Hanson, C. M. (2005). *Advanced practice nursing: An integrative approach* (3rd ed.). St. Louis, MO: Elsevier Saunders.

Matuson, R. C. (2011). *Suddenly in charge: Managing up, managing down, succeeding all around.* Boston, MA: Nicholas Brealey.

McNichol, J. (2013). Manage up: Use these six tips to cultivate a healthy working relationship with your boss. *American Speech-Language-Hearing Association Leader, 18*(10), 28–29.

Pearce, C. (2007). Ten steps to managing your boss. *Nursing Management, 14*(3), 21.

Scott, D. E. (2007). Collaboration with your boss: Strategic skills for professional nurses. *South Carolina Nurse, 14*(1), 21.

Sparacino, P. S. A., Cooper, D. M., & Minarik, P. A. (1990). *The clinical nurse specialist: Implementation and impact.* Norwalk, CT: Appleton & Lange.

Tulgan, B. (2010). *It's okay to manage your boss: The first step-by-step program for making the best of your most important relationship at work.* San Francisco, CA: Jossey-Bass.

PART II

MOVING FORWARD

CHAPTER 5

Learning the Ropes: Orientation

RUTHANN B. ZAFIAN

BE PROACTIVE: ASK FOR WHAT YOU WANT DURING YOUR ORIENTATION AND BEYOND

How exciting! You've accepted or are about to accept your first job as a clinical nurse specialist (CNS). Start creating opportunities for success the moment you accept the job. Now is the time to start negotiating your orientation so you meet the people you need to know to begin analyzing the culture of your new work environment. It doesn't matter whether you're a novice or an experienced CNS, whether you're new to the institution or have worked there for years. You know your strengths and challenges. You know what knowledge and skill you bring to the table. You know your learning needs and learning style. So be proactive right from the start and ask for what you need in your orientation while also taking the time to teach others about all you have to offer. This is the time when your schedule will be the most flexible, before you get caught up in assignments, meetings, and clinical consultations. So take full advantage of it and learn everything you can.

THE VALUE OF GENERIC ORIENTATION CLASSES

You may be required to attend hospital-wide, generic, and nursing department orientation programs, along with a variety of other hospital employees including the staff nurses. Though you may feel some of these classes are very basic, unnecessary, and not directly applicable to your work, don't fight it. There will be some pearls of information that you will find useful in some manner. Some of these classes are required by state or federal agencies, and all of them will afford you the opportunity to experience the orientation programs that are provided for new staff nurses. You need to know what they are being taught if you hope to influence the system in the nursing/nursing practice sphere (National Association of Clinical Nurse Specialists [NACNS], 2004). This is also an opportunity to start evaluating the quality of information provided to new nurses and the relationship that the Nursing Department has with other departments.

SO, WHAT IS A CNS? WHAT EXACTLY DO YOU DO?

You will be asked: "What does a CNS do?" So you'd better be prepared to answer that question with a succinct but informative explanation. This may be your first opportunity to establish relationships with colleagues and staff members. These first-impression meetings are important. Memorize your standard CNS statement, but your delivery may vary based on who asks the question. If a physician or an administrator were to ask the question, I'd say something like: "My focus is on optimizing clinical practice, patient outcomes, and staff knowledge. I do this by helping nurses and other health care providers understand and use evidence to improve nursing practice. I also focus on improving intra- and interdepartmental systems using appreciative inquiry, root cause analysis, change theory, and other quality improvement techniques."

If a staff nurse asked me the question, I'd say: "I'm here to make it as easy as possible for you to provide excellent patient and family care. I'll do this by making sure you have the information and knowledge you need. If you want to learn a new procedure, I can help. If you need information about a patient's diagnosis that you haven't seen before, I can help. I'll also be your advocate. I believe your voice needs to be heard when new equipment or processes are being evaluated. But first I need to know what you think about your work here, what works well, and what needs improvement. I need you to teach me, so I can help you."

How would you answer this question? However you choose to deliver your message, make sure you have it on the tip of your tongue because you will be asked that question over and over. Some CNSs add a descriptive statement to the auto-signature that appears at the end of all of their e-mails or have a statement printed on the back of their business cards. The point is, you should never pass up the opportunity to help others understand the role and value of the CNS.

When I took on my first job as a CNS, I met the chief of cardiac surgery. As I anticipated, he asked me the "What's a CNS?" question. I explained my role, but he looked perplexed. Then he asked, "So, do I now have to go to you when I'm having trouble finding a bed for my patient?" I paused, pretended to wipe sweat from my brow, and said, "Thankfully, no. That's not my role." Be prepared for questions such as these by anticipating the interests and issues that are important to the person with whom you'll be meeting. Though I was not the person in charge of bed assignments, I quickly assured the chief of service that I would help optimize nursing care, system efficiencies, and patient outcomes so that patients move from the intensive care unit (ICU) to telemetry to discharge in a timely and efficient manner. Essentially, I would help optimize patient throughput so beds would be available for the next surgical case. He nodded and seemed satisfied with that answer.

You also need to get used to saying, "I don't know, but I'll find out and get back to you." As a novice in the CNS role and perhaps a novice to the institution, you may find yourself in the uncomfortable position of being asked one or several questions during these encounters, the answers to which you may have no idea. But that's okay. No one expects you to have all the answers. They will, however, expect that you will follow through and be 100% reliable. So if you say, "I'll get back to you," make sure to keep your promise. You may also get stumped by some of the questions you'll be asked. When I was orienting to my first job as a CNS, I met with the chief of trauma services. He asked me, "What's your philosophy of nursing?" I never expected that question. It really took me by surprise. I'm sure I gave him the "deer in the headlights" look for at least 5 seconds, but then I regained some of my composure. I remember mumbling something about incorporating aspects of several nursing models into my approach to clinical practice. Today, I would be much better prepared.

Try to end each one of these introductory meetings with two questions: "If I have a question about something that involves your department, may I contact you or whom would you like me to call?" You may also want to say "Now that you know a bit about my role, can you think of projects already in progress or coming up in the future where I may be of help?"

FIND YOURSELF A MENTOR

Make sure to spend a few hours shadowing other CNSs who work in your hospital. It's important to see how they enact the role and to establish these relationships with your peers. Many times, these CNSs will be your greatest allies and sources of information about the inner workings and politics of the institution. When you meet with the other CNSs, ask how they quantify and qualify their work. If the CNSs in your hospital meet regularly to share information, support one another's work, or do group projects, make sure you join and attend these meetings.

Because even the most pro-CNS institutions employ a limited number of CNSs, and sometimes only one per specialty, it's easy to feel isolated. Make contact and stay in touch with your peers. Seek out one or more of these CNSs as your mentor. If you are the only CNS at your institution, consider someone in nursing education or administration as your mentor. The person you choose as your mentor should be someone who is open to a mentoring relationship with you, someone whom you can trust and communicate with easily. This person should be someone who also has leadership or operational qualities you admire. Even if that CNS works in a completely different specialty area of nursing, that CNS can help you acclimate to your new role.

Also, try to find out if there is a regional CNS group that meets regularly in your area. Never underestimate the power of networking. Contact with these other CNSs is especially important if you are the only CNS at your institution. You'll need the support of people who understand the unique and challenging role of the CNS. It's very interesting to speak with CNSs from other institutions and compare and contrast the implementation of their roles. You may be surprised to learn how many projects and issues you have in common. Share your ideas freely and borrow great ideas whenever you can as long as you give credit where the credit is due. Join an online listserve group for CNSs. You'll have the opportunity to connect with CNSs all over the United States and beyond. Be sure to stay in touch with colleagues and speakers you meet at conferences and share best practice ideas.

GET TO KNOW YOUR CUSTOMERS

Build in plenty of time to shadow some of the staff nurses on all shifts with whom you will be working. You need time to make sure you get to know them, their needs, and concerns. They in turn need time to get comfortable with you. Though CNS job descriptions vary from institution to institution, almost all call for spending a considerable amount of time working within the patient/client and nursing/nursing practice spheres of influence (NACNS, 2004). So working with staff during your orientation will be very valuable to your future success. As you spend time observing and getting to know the staff nurses with whom you'll be working, simply offer your assistance. Use humor and remain nononfrontational, even when challenged with skeptical or rude remarks. When I started at my current job, I asked one ICU nurse how I could help her. She smirked and replied: "So are you ready to get your hands dirty?" I winked and responded: "Sure, at least to get my gloves dirty." Keep in mind that famous quote from Theodore Roosevelt, "No one cares how much you know until they know how much you care" (Rierson, 2014). It still rings true today. If you are helpful and listen well, the nurses will start to trust you. They will seek you out, ask you questions, and be open to learning from you.

"SEEK FIRST TO UNDERSTAND, THEN TO BE UNDERSTOOD"

You may be very eager to get in and prove yourself, make a difference, and show people what you know. But when you are new to the CNS role, I suggest you tread very lightly at first. These first encounters with the staff nurses are your one and only chance for first impressions. Your demeanor needs to be friendly and that of a learner. Keep this motto from Stephen Covey (2004) in mind: "Seek first to understand, then to be understood." In reality, you will learn as much from the staff nurses as they will learn from you. If nurses are to eventually learn from you, they will first need to feel emotionally safe around you. If you are speaking with a nurse or other colleague and you start to sense that the person does not feel safe, it is in your best interest to change tactics to help the other feel safe again (Patterson, Grenny, McMillan, & Switzler, 2002). You need to understand and show respect for the nurse's strengths and frustrations. You may see behaviors and styles of practice that you feel need to be improved upon, but when you are new to the CNS role, avoid being critical until you understand these important customers better. Of course, if you see unsafe practice, you'll need to step in immediately, but your approach in these situations is key to future success. Understand that some folks will be intimidated by you or will resent you before they even meet you. This is not unusual in some staff nurses and even some nurse managers who do not have the degree(s), experience, or credentials that you have. Again, tread lightly and help these colleagues to feel safe around you. Show appreciation for the knowledge and experience that these nurses bring to the table, and those barriers to collaboration will disappear eventually.

If you're in a situation where you are transitioning from the role of staff nurse to CNS in the same organization or within the same unit or service, be assertive and set limits as you transition to your new role. You may be tempted to do many of the things you did as a staff nurse because that is your comfort zone. Others may have difficulty understanding your nonclinical responsibilities and even expect that you will supplement staffing numbers. In time you will find a new comfort zone in the role of the CNS. Do not allow staff or managers to think of you as a per diem staff member. You certainly want staff nurses to request clinical consultations with you and ask for your help at the bedside, but it is not your job to replace the nurse at the bedside. I have heard of programs that require CNSs to provide direct care and take a staff assignment for a predetermined set of days or hours each month. The rationale is to ensure you are able to maintain your clinical proficiency. Though I do not believe this is the best use of the CNS, if you agree to this when you are hired into the role, go with it, but resist being used as a supplemental staff member on other days. You have very important work to do beyond direct patient care. That work requires a flexible schedule for meetings, literature reviews, research, quality improvement work, and consultations with members of the multidisciplinary health care team.

AVOID ROLE AMBIGUITY

Request weekly meetings with your director/supervisor for at least the first month or two, then continue to meet at least monthly during your tenure. This is essential to stay focused, keep your priorities in line with that of your department or institution, and avoid role ambiguity. Role ambiguity arises when the post holder and/or other stakeholders are unclear or hold different conceptions of the role (Jones, 2005). The role of the CNS overlaps somewhat and also complements the roles of many other health care team members: the manager, the educator, and the nurse practitioner. If the CNS is unclear about his or her role within the organization, then the CNS will not be able to present himself or herself confidently and will falter during this critical transition time. Your director or supervisor is the person with whom you need to negotiate the expectations of your role. You will also need the support of your director or supervisor to reinforce that description and differentiation of your role to others on the team. When I began my role as a cardiovascular CNS, one of our nurse educators asked me to explain the difference between the roles of the CNS and the nurse educator. We had a nice discussion about the differences and the areas where our roles might overlap. She and I have always worked well together and have had no difficulties with role clarity. However, I remember speaking to my director about that discussion between the nurse educator and myself and was surprised at the alarm that sounded in her voice as she recounted the role ambiguity problems that had plagued the person who was in the cardiovascular CNS role before me. My director was determined not to allow that to become a problem again and set about making sure I, along with others on the team, knew what her role expectations were (for all of us).

As stated, you may be expected to spend a certain number of hours each week or month providing direct patient care to maintain your clinical skills. Others may expect you to keep a record of your time and activities to ensure you are allocating enough of your time to being available to the staff. Make sure you discuss these role expectations with your director early in your orientation. If possible, use technology to your advantage. Set up databases, spreadsheets, or Word documents to track your projects and goals. You may even want to adopt a tool developed by another CNS to record and report your contributions in the workplace (Colwill et al., 2014). I was able to have the information systems department at my hospital build a feature into our computer order-entry system where anyone on staff could order a CNS consult with me regarding a specific patient by just a few clicks of the computer mouse. This gives the nursing staff an easy way to initiate consults with me. Since I cover several different inpatient units, I also find it very helpful at the end of the year to run reports from this system that spell out the number of consults I get from each unit, the reason for the consult, and who initiated the consult. As health care dollars shrink, more and more CNSs will have to justify their worth to their institutions. A report demonstrating the links between project outcomes and activities will help administrators understand your worth even if your position is not revenue generating (Fulton, 2013).

You can explore other ways that the technology available in your institution might be helpful to you. For instance, does your hospital have an electronic incident reporting system? Whether the system for these reports is paper or electronic, is it possible for you to have access to the reports? It will help you identify learning needs and issues that need further investigation. If you have e-mail and Internet access in your office, be sure to sign up to automatically receive e-newsletters from organizations associated with your work, such as your state hospital association or other specific nursing organizations such as the NACNS. I subscribe to several e-newsletters and read them regularly. Keeping current on issues and research in your specialty is essential.

Access to information is crucial to your success as a CNS. Your director needs to understand that you need to be kept informed about a wide variety of issues affecting your areas. This includes information specific to the role and functions of managers. You may not be involved in the decisions surrounding these issues, but it is essential that you are aware of issues that may stress the staff or the patients with whom you work. You may need to present a persuasive argument to achieve this. Your director needs to know the benefits of keeping you in the loop. It is important that he or she trusts your discretion regarding sensitive topics and also that you understand the boundaries of your input and influence. If you are unsure whether the information being shared with you is confidential or ready for wider distribution, be sure to ask. Also, don't be afraid to ask to be included on projects or committees that are of interest to you. There will be times when you learn about a new initiative that you find objectionable. You may want to ask if the topic is negotiable before sharing your objections to the plan with your director. For example, at my particular worksite, for several years we avoided hiring graduate nurses (GNs) into the critical care areas, but because of staffing shortages, management felt it was necessary to allow GNs this option. When I was informed about this, my first question to the director was, "Is this a done deal or are you asking for my opinion about the plan?" I was told this was a done deal, so in spite of my significant reservations about the plan, my response was to advise the director about what would be needed to successfully support the new ICU GNs to achieve competency, staff satisfaction, retention, and maintain patient safety.

As you and your director come to a consensus about your role, begin to develop SMART goals (Donahue, 2007). You should be able to start formulating such goals about a month or two after you've started and have begun to understand the priorities within your service line. SMART is an acronym for (S) specific, (M) measurable, (A) attainable, (R) realistic, and (T) tangible or timely (Donahue, 2007). An example of a poorly worded goal is: "I will improve the quality of hand-off reports within my service line." A better goal might be: "By the end of this month, I will complete a survey of the ICU staff members regarding the issues surrounding hand-off report quality and develop a plan of action." If your institution used dashboards to establish and track goals, ensure your goals are aligned accordingly.

There is one other topic you may want to discuss with your director. If there was a CNS in your position previously, it is important for you to understand his or her legacy. Was that person well liked and successful, or was that person unsuccessful in the role and why? You may encounter more opposition from staff members if that last CNS was unable to win the respect of the staff or leadership team. If the previous CNS was well liked, I would ask staff members what it was that made that CNS successful. Liked or disliked, the "ghosts of CNSs past" may haunt you, but you will be more prepared to deal with this legacy if you understand the impressions that were left behind.

BUILD A STRONG AND DIVERSE NETWORK OF PROFESSIONAL CONTACTS

You'll need to determine who are your primary and secondary customers. Some will be obvious, such as those within your own service line: your director, the nurse manager(s), the nurse educator(s), physicians, advanced practice nurses, physician assistants, and staff nurses. Others may not be so obvious: the manager of the respiratory therapists, the manager of medical records, and so forth. Remember you are entering a role where you will need to negotiate within all three CNS spheres of influence (NACNS, 2004). Your work in the organizational/systems spheres will require your ability to influence decisions well beyond your service line. It's important that you spend time learning about the needs of each of these customers. Learn what your primary customers' needs or wants are, and make those your first projects. Some will have absolutely no idea what to do with you, and others will have extensive ideas.

Your relationship with the nurse manager(s) with whom you'll be working most closely can make or break you. Any change process you want to move forward that involves staff nurses will be in jeopardy unless you have the visible support of the nurse/unit manager, the person with line authority. CNS job descriptions vary greatly from person to person and from institution to institution, but one variable remains fairly constant. Every CNS is a change agent, and many CNSs work without direct line authority. So your professional network and alliances will be vital to your ability to move agendas forward. I find face-to-face meetings much more productive than phone conversations or e-mails, especially when the subject matter might be controversial. I use e-mail for updates and "FYIs" and for setting up meetings, but if topics need to be discussed in depth and decisions made, I prefer meeting directly with the person or persons involved.

Once you've met most of your primary customers, arrange introductory meetings with folks outside your immediate service line and outside the Department of Nursing; for example, respiratory therapy, pharmacy, purchasing, library, quality management, and physician chiefs of service, medical records, information technology services, the emergency department, and so. Again, these folks may be very helpful as you start working on house-wide projects or teams. Health care is changing so rapidly these days. Your conversations with these managers and practitioners from other departments will help you broaden your perspective and understand the business of health care including its constraints (Beglinger, 2014). When you attend meetings, if there is anyone in the room whom you haven't met before, walk right up and introduce yourself. Build yourself a reputation for being friendly, assertive, and confident (Sullivan, 2013).

RESERVE TIME FOR REFLECTION

It's tough being a novice again, but anytime you take on a new role or a new job you'll return to being a novice for a while. The good news is that, because you have some experience behind you and the benefits of your graduate education, you'll probably advance out of the novice stage fairly quickly. Still, you may not feel completely comfortable with your new role for a full year. This is a new and expanded role for you. The politics of the CNS role can be very challenging and the stress can wear you down. It's important to take time every day to decompress, reflect, and renew. How? That's for you to decide. Whether it's a walk outside at lunchtime or a few minutes in your office with your favorite music playing, make sure you find some time for you. These quiet moments are necessary to find clarity and allow innovative thinking. This is key for your future success.

It may be helpful to keep in contact with some of your graduate school professors or those who graduated from the CNS program with you. Support each other and share your experiences. They may be dealing with or have dealt with similar challenging situations and have some pearls of wisdom for you. The benefits of building a large, strong foundation of professional contacts should not be underestimated.

RELATIONSHIPS

I can't overemphasize that the strength of your relationships with your director and your customers is your greatest asset. Develop an ever-present "I'm here to help" attitude and check your ego at the door. It may take a while before you're given responsibility for projects or committee work. Be patient and prove your ability with whatever projects come your way. The projects you are most interested in will come in time if you do well with the assignments that are handed to you. It's all about putting the patients and families first and mentoring other health care professionals and workers to do the same. Just as with any job, there will be days when you leave work feeling as if you've really made a positive impact and other days where you feel frustrated and dejected. Find constructive outlets for your own frustrations at the job and always try to maintain a cool head and a professional demeanor. Make great first impressions and then work to maintain these relationships. This approach will truly take you far.

SUMMARY

1. Be proactive: Ask for what you want during your orientation.
2. Attend the generic orientation program and learn everything you can from it.
3. Memorize your CNS role description statement and share it with everyone who will listen.
4. Find a mentor: Shadow other CNSs.
5. Get to know your primary customers and help them feel safe around you.

6. "Seek first to understand, then to be understood" (Covey, 2004).
7. Avoid role ambiguity and develop SMART goals.
8. Build a strong and diverse network of professional contacts.
9. Take time every day to decompress, reflect, and renew.
10. Maintain the strong relationships you've established with your peers and customers.

REFERENCES

Beglinger, J. (2014). Clinical nurse specialists: Choosing to lead in an era of reform. *Clinical Nurse Specialist, 28*, 81–82.

Colwill, J., O'Rourke, C., Booher, L., Soat, M., Solomon, D., & Albert, N. (2014). Capture of knowledge work of clinical nurse specialists using a role tracking tool. *Clinical Nurse Specialist, 28*, 323–331.

Covey, S. (2004). *7 habits of highly successful people: 15th anniversary edition*. New York, NY: Simon & Schuster.

Donahue, G. (2007). *Top achievement: Creating S.M.A.R.T goals*. Retrieved from http://www.topachievement.com/smart

Fulton, J. (2013). Making outcomes of clinical nurse specialist practice visible. *Clinical Nurse Specialist, 27*, 5–6.

Jones, M. L. (2005). Role development and effective practice in specialist and advanced practice roles in acute hospital setting: Systematic review and meta-synthesis. *Journal of Advanced Nursing, 49*(2), 191–209.

National Association of Clinical Nurse Specialists (NACNS). (2004). *Statement on clinical nurse specialist practice and education* (2nd ed.). Harrisburg, PA: Author.

Patterson, K., Grenny, J., McMillan, R., & Switzler, A. (2002). *Crucial conversations: Tools for talking when stakes are high*. New York, NY: McGraw-Hill.

Rierson, R. (2014, November 9). *20 Inspirational Theodore Roosevelt quotes*. Retrieved from http://www.doseofleadersip.com

Sullivan, E. J. (2013). *Becoming influential: A guide for nurses*. Upper Saddle River, NJ: Prentice-Hall.

CHAPTER 6

Establishing Credibility

RUTH VAN GERPEN

Gloria has recently completed her master's in nursing program as a clinical nurse specialist (CNS) and has accepted a CNS position at a medical center in her community. Prior to graduation, Gloria worked as an evening charge nurse at another hospital for 3 years since completing her BSN degree. She is excited about starting a new job but is apprehensive about the staff accepting her as a CNS. She wonders to herself, "Do I know enough to do this job?"

Kate, a classmate of Gloria's, has the same concerns. Kate has worked as a staff nurse at the community hospital for 15 years before pursuing her dream of becoming a CNS. The director of nursing offered Kate a position as a CNS in the hospital following graduation. She's worried that her coworkers won't take her seriously in her new role. Gloria and Kate both recognize the importance of establishing credibility in their new roles.

The root of the word credibility is *credo*, which means "I believe" in Latin (Lopez, 2010). *Merriam-Webster* defines "credible" as capable of being believed, believable, and trustworthy. Credibility requires clinical expertise, the thoughtful application of knowledge, and the demonstration of behaviors that create a reputation of trustworthiness. When Kouzes and Posner (1993) asked people to define credibility in behavioral terms, "the most frequent response was 'they do what they say they will do,' 'they practice what they preach,' 'they walk the talk,' and 'their actions are consistent with their words'" (p. 47).

DiSabatino Smith (2005) found that RNs identify work ethic, expertise, and character as attributes of clinical credibility. Previous research outside of nursing has identified "expertise" and "trustworthiness" as attributes of credibility. The attribute of "work ethic" emerged as an attribute unique to nursing. In her study, RNs with a good work ethic were described as those who have organizational skills; pay attention to detail; are very thorough, efficient, follow through, and do not let things "fall through the cracks"; are well prepared, able to manage any patient/family situation, and are solution-oriented, hard working, willing to help other coworkers; and are willing to go the extra mile to get the job done.

The credibility foundation is built brick by brick. It is earned over time and sustained through hard work. A solid foundation of personal credibility is necessary for the CNS to generate confidence, gain commitment from others, and achieve desired patient outcomes or organizational goals and objectives.

ESTABLISHING CREDIBLE RELATIONSHIPS

Gloria is excited about her new job at the medical center but isn't sure where to start. To facilitate her transition (integration) to the CNS role, Gloria's supervisor asked Helen, an experienced CNS at the medical center, to be Gloria's "buddy." In addition, Gloria's supervisor also developed a structured orientation plan for her. Whether new or experienced, the CNS needs the time and opportunity to become acquainted with the organizational structure, mission, policies, and procedures of the institution. Included in Gloria's orientation are appointments with key individuals. It is important for Gloria to establish a credible relationship with the formal and informal leaders in the organization to accomplish the desired patient care outcomes. These meetings are a first step, providing Gloria with an opportunity to understand each person's responsibilities and explain her role as a CNS and how she can be a valuable resource. These individuals may vary based on departmental structures and specific job descriptions and responsibilities:

- Nursing administrators
- Physicians
- Nurse managers/assistant nurse managers
- Unit charge nurses, preceptors
- Administrative supervisors
- Interdisciplinary team members: pharmacists, chaplains, dieticians, therapists
- CNS colleagues
- Nurse educators
- Quality improvement/quality assurance staff
- Data analysts

Prior to the appointments, Helen helped Gloria understand the "lay of the land" in the organization: the administrative reporting structure, departmental relationships, and whom to call. Helen commented that one of the most difficult things when she started her job was deciphering the organizational process for implementing practice changes. She shared the following example with Gloria. One of the first practices in need of change was implementation of the evidence-based recommendations for safe handling of hazardous drugs. At the suggestion of her buddy, Helen initially visited with the safety officer; directors of pharmacy, environmental services, and central supply; and nurse managers of oncology and critical care. She not only received support for the practice change but also received differing opinions of the sequence of steps necessary for implementation and whether final approval belonged to the safety officer, the director of nursing, or the nursing practice committee. Instead of trying to determine the process herself, Helen invited the key individuals to a meeting and together they identified the necessary changes, the sequence for implementation, and who had final approval. Helen commented that, because of her approach, she felt she had begun to gain the trust of several leaders in the organization.

FROM STAFF NURSE CREDIBLE TO EXPERT CREDIBLE: DEALING WITH CHALLENGERS

Despite her years of experience as an RN prior to becoming a CNS, Kate found herself unprepared for her feelings of inadequacy when being questioned by staff about a patient care issue outside her area of expertise. Now that she was the specialist, the staff teasingly commented she should know everything. Kate admitted she thought she should know the answer because a CNS is the expert. After a particularly difficult week, Kate began to wonder if she really belonged in this position. Fortunately, Kate shared her doubts with her supervisor, who reassured her that these feelings are normal, especially in a new role or a new job. She also told Kate that the longer she stays in her CNS role and develops more expertise and knowledge, the less often she will experience these feelings of doubt and inadequacy.

The term *imposter phenomenon* has been used throughout psychology and sociology literature to describe individuals who feel as if they are imposters in their chosen profession. Often, it is a transient experience associated with specific situations such as starting a new job or moving into a new role (Harvey & Katz, 1985). Clinical symptoms associated with this phenomenon are generalized anxiety, lack of self-confidence, depression, and frustration related to an inability to meet a self-imposed standard of achievement (Clance & Imes, 1978). Arena and Page (1992) believe that a form of the imposter phenomenon is inherent in the CNS role. It is characterized by feelings of inadequacy and of constantly being tested, no matter how confident or self-secure the CNS feels. Questioning whether he or she belongs in the position may become all-encompassing and should be expected with a new role. These feelings may resurface when a change occurs in the role. If these symptoms extend into the CNS's personal life, the person may be experiencing the full effects of the phenomenon.

To help ease the feelings of doubt, Kate and her supervisor identified several strategies she can implement:

- Find a CNS mentor with whom Kate can share her feelings and who will help Kate reestablish her self-confidence.
- Identify supportive colleagues at work who are willing to share their knowledge and expertise.
- Continue to provide direct patient care on a regular basis to maintain and strengthen clinical skills and develop clinical competence in weak areas.

- Develop a personal library by gathering and maintaining current information on relevant clinical topics. Kate can use the information to answer clinical questions from staff or post copies of journal articles pertinent to the unit's patient population.
- Name a difference she has made to a patient, family, staff member, or colleague every day.

Kate's first step was to contact Brenda, a CNS at another hospital in town. Brenda, a CNS for 5 years, was delighted when Kate asked for her help and guidance. She shared with Kate her initial challenge of working with a nurse manager who felt threatened by her involvement and therefore didn't want any CNS help on the unit. Kate admitted she was grateful that this hadn't been a problem for her, but was intrigued to learn how Brenda dealt with this challenge. Brenda shared that she had taken the advice of her mentor, who suggested she focus on the units where her help was wanted, not stress over the manager who didn't understand the CNS role. Within a year, the skeptical nurse manager asked Brenda for her help. She had heard from several other nurse managers that Brenda had been helpful in working with staff to identify appropriate solutions to specific clinical practice issues and had been a valuable clinical role model and mentor for new nurses in their clinical areas.

DEMONSTRATING CREDIBILITY

After several months, Brenda invited Kate to attend a quarterly CNS networking meeting attended by CNSs from surrounding communities. At the meeting, Kate saw Gloria and asked how she was enjoying her new job. Gloria shared her struggles with being new in an organization: getting acquainted with key individuals, learning the organizational structure, and gaining the trust of the nursing staff. Kate commented that her struggles have surprised her. She thought the transition to CNS would be easy, as she was familiar with the organization and the nursing staff. She didn't expect to be questioned about her knowledge and challenged about ulterior motives, such as being after the nurse manager's job.

Brenda introduced Kate and Gloria and asked the other CNSs to share a strategy or personal example of what they did as new CNSs to gain the confidence and trust of others and gain credibility. The CNSs in attendance were eager to share their suggestions, because as one nurse commented, "We've all been there at least once." Suggested strategies included:

- Schedule time for direct patient care and don't cancel. Working as staff and caring for patients in difficult situations provide an opportunity to prove your skills as a nurse and demonstrate your value as a useful resource.
- Work an off-shift periodically to demonstrate competence, serve as a role model, and provide opportunity for interaction and problem solving

with evening and night staff. It also allows the CNS to observe actual implementation of nursing processes and procedures.

- Attend shift report and team meetings and/or conduct patient-centered rounds, focusing on patient and family needs. Discuss and problem-solve issues identified during report or rounds with the nursing staff.
- Participate in staff meetings and offer to present a short educational program on a topic identified through a needs assessment.
- Offer to provide clinical expertise during a root cause analysis process or investigation of an unexpected patient outcome.
- Assist nurse educators or nurse managers with staff competencies or a hospital-wide education day.
- Write a brief article on a relevant clinical topic for a nursing unit or nursing department newsletter.

One strategy that received resounding agreement was the importance of maintaining a regular presence in the clinical nursing areas. This also allows the CNS to promote his or her area of expertise. Joan shared her experience to illustrate this point. As a CNS with extensive pain management experience, Joan struggled with getting the staff to utilize her expertise. One day during patient rounds, Joan identified a patient with inadequate postoperative pain control despite the efforts of the nursing staff. During her patient interview and assessment, Joan discovered the patient had been taking a long-acting opioid for the past year due to a chronic pain condition. On admission, the long-acting opioid had not been continued, and the amount of IV analgesic the patient was receiving for postoperative pain control was less than the patient had been taking preoperatively, accounting for the inadequate pain management. Joan shared her findings and recommendations with the staff nurse and the physician. During rounds the next day, the patient told Joan his pain was much better and he had been able to get some sleep during the night. Seeing Joan on the unit, a staff nurse asked her to see another patient about pain management. Several days later, Joan also received a consult request from the physician to see a patient for pain control suggestions. Joan firmly believes her constant visibility made the difference in laying the foundation for establishing her credibility as a CNS.

Credibility is about being believed, being competent, having a good work ethic, and being trustworthy. It provides the foundation for the CNS to generate confidence, gain commitment from others, and achieve desired patient outcomes or organizational goals and objectives. Credibility does make a difference.

REFERENCES

Arena, D. M., & Page, N. E. (1992). The imposter phenomenon in the clinical nurse specialist role. *Image: Journal of Nursing Scholarship, 24*(2), 121–125.

Clance, P. R., & Imes, S. A. (1978). The imposter phenomenon in high achieving women: Dynamics and therapeutic intervention. *Psychotherapy: Theory, Research and Practice, 15*(3), 241–246.

DiSabatino Smith, C. (2005). Identifying attributes of clinical credibility in registered nurses. *Nursing Administration Quarterly, 29*(2), 188–191.

Harvey, J. C., & Katz, C. (1985). *If I'm so successful, why do I feel like a fake? The imposter phenomenon.* New York, NY: St. Martin's Press.

Kouzes, J. M., & Posner, B. Z. (1993). *Credibility: How leaders gain and lose it, why people demand it.* San Francisco, CA: Jossey-Bass.

Lopez, A. (2010). *The legacy leader.* Mustang, OK: Tate Publishing Enterprises LLC.

CHAPTER 7

Prioritizing: Avoiding Overcommitment and Underachievement

KATIE BRUSH

Welcome to a new role. Welcome to the world of the clinical nurse specialist (CNS). Welcome to the world of time management. Time management is essential to avoiding overcommitment, which is the slippery slope toward underachievement. The first year of CNS practice can be frustrating due to learning to juggle multiple competing demands and divergent responsibilities. Hopefully, this chapter gives you some tips on achieving balance and avoiding the pitfalls of this new practice.

A new CNS is presented with many opportunities to make a difference such as introducing evidence-based practice, leading performance improvement, updating procedures—initiatives aimed at improving patient care and outcomes. A new CNS is eager to become involved and demonstrate new skills. In the beginning, it may seem as though there is a massive amount of work to do. With so many opportunities, a novice CNS is vulnerable to overcommitment, thus time management becomes critical from the very beginning. Most new CNSs have worked as staff nurses before going to graduate school. Staff nurse work has rather defined boundaries—the schedule is fixed, days and times determined, the patient assignment is clear, and when the shift is over, a staff nurse goes home. Not so for the CNS. A typical new CNS is not well prepared to manage multiple competing demands at the system level. Sure, graduate school had numerous deadlines and meeting the demands of multiple assignments may have been challenging; however, the difference is that now *you*, the CNS, participate in determining the assignment. Many new CNSs underestimate the amount of time and energy needed to develop, implement, evaluate, revise, monitor, and continuously support unit-level or system-level projects. Avoid believing you can leap tall buildings in a single bound. It's not true for anyone, and for a novice it is a sure way to fail.

There will always be colleagues, staff, and bosses ready to fill the plate of the new CNS. It is a great honor for the new CNS to be trusted enough to be asked to take on important projects. Be cautious; start small. Select projects where the time to completion is delimited and the chance of success is high. Too many projects (projects that are complex or projects that may take months or years to complete) will not give a new CNS the gratification and confidence that success builds. Despite coursework, no matter how helpful, role-related culture shock is present from the moment you enter the work world as a new CNS. Before saying yes to an assignment, ask yourself: "Am I up to this challenge? Is this the best project for me at this time? Can I succeed?" Remember to start small and build a record of successes.

The boss can help you prioritize. Discuss your goals with the boss and determine the boss's goals for you. The negotiation process between the two of you should take into account your level of experience. If the boss has never worked with a CNS, or worked with CNSs in roles not including competencies in the three spheres—patient, nurses/nursing practice, and system—you may also need to negotiate the focus of your role. CNSs eager to please may be inclined to take on any project assigned by the boss. Negotiate! Be prepared to discuss how the new project fits into your current priorities. Ask the boss: "What would you like me to give up in order to take this on?" Asked respectfully in the context of prioritizing your work, it is not insubordination. Prioritizing with the boss helps you to control your workload. Discuss current projects and assignments, progress toward completion, and rationale for ongoing involvement. The boss may have an entirely different idea. Listen to the boss's viewpoint. The ability to compromise and listen to each other is essential. But don't negotiate away all the things you enjoy. The job will become drudgery unless you are able to keep some things that you value most in your list of priorities. For example, if you enjoy making rounds in the intensive care unit to "case find" patient problems, don't eliminate this completely to take on a major project that will remove you from the unit for months. Compromise. You might reduce your rounds from daily to three times a week and ask for an assistant or cochair for the project.

THE NURSING STAFF

As a new CNS, you must meet the staff—nurses, therapists, clerks, housekeepers, and others who work in your specialty area. Learn their names, years of experience, type of assignments they prefer. Observe practice and consider spending time orienting yourself to the staff nurse role in the specialty setting. Remind staff that you will not be very effective in helping them with patient care if you don't understand patient care in the unit. Be clear that you are not orienting so you can fill in for vacations, lunch assignments, or unanticipated absences. You are learning the role so you can appreciate their perspectives and understand their challenges and opportunities. Orientation is time limited. Let the staff know the time—a couple of weeks should be adequate to learn the staff nurse role. Depending on your familiarity with the unit or type of care setting, more or less time for orientation may be needed.

While orienting yourself, ask the staff about things they would change if they could. Listen to what issues each staff member identifies as problems.

Keep a list, and review it for similarities between staff members. Create categories of ideas that you may want to address in the future. Prioritize the ideas. Start small. Nothing breeds success like fixing a relatively simple problem that has irritated staff for a prolonged time. It may be a problem that you would never have considered until the staff pointed it out. You will win the staff's trust when you successfully address their problems.

COLLEAGUES

Colleagues can be your best allies. They can help you to sort out some of your big and small questions. Learn from others' experiences and value stories for the lessons they teach. Spend time with other junior colleagues and see how they are managing. Keep your eyes and ears open. Watch for habits that some colleagues may have developed that you want to avoid, such as spending late nights working on projects, or being involved in so many things that they are ineffective. Notice how others manage time well and make respected contributions. Try to emulate the good work habits and avoid the pitfalls. A successful CNS has often spent years learning to stay focused, manage time, prioritize projects, and avoid overcommitment. Ask experienced CNSs to share secrets to prioritizing tasks and managing time.

FLYING UNDER THE RADAR

Role success means being effective. You cannot be effective if you are stretched too thin. A new CNS should ascribe to the notion of "flying under the radar," or, in other words, keeping a low profile. Don't volunteer for every committee, program, project, and work group. Be selective. Spend most of your time listening. Give yourself time to learn the organizational culture. Begin by focusing your efforts on staff and patient care. There will be pressure to join in the projects involving the global arena. Listen to the concerns, but don't offer your time. Learn the politics. You are a "can do" professional, but avoid the desire to do everything for everyone.

Your arrival has been anxiously awaited and productivity anticipated. Most likely, many individuals will have preconceived ideas of your role and have formulated goals. Others may want to assign projects and committee work to you. In a meeting with a group of your peers, or with any group that is interested in a new endeavor, you do *not* need to jump in—don't be the first to volunteer. Suffer through the uncomfortable silences that arise in the group and wait for a more experienced person to volunteer. You are eager to please and prove your abilities, but jumping in is a sure way to becoming overcommitted and ineffective. If the project is complex, you may feel overwhelmed. This feeling is a good indication that the project is something you should avoid. If it becomes necessary to take on the new project, ask for another, more senior, CNS to work with you.

It is an honor to be asked to contribute. The feeling of being needed is gratifying. The idea that your opinion is important can be terrifying and thrilling at the same time. Set priorities that will most benefit your cohort of patients, whether through the staff or the system. Work on a few value-added projects. Choose opportunities that will have the greatest effect on improvement in patient care in your area(s).

Carve out a niche in your area of expertise within your first years of practice by carefully selecting problems and projects that build your reputation of success. Become the "go to" person for one or two patient care issues. Soon you will be receiving requests to consult on problems related to your niche specialty focus, which will give you more insight into the organization. The more knowledge you gain about your specialty area within the organization, the more you will be able to contribute.

TIME MANAGEMENT

Maybe you are a great planner, scheduler, and finisher, or maybe you have great coordination skills. If this is true of you, keep it up. If not, find ways to be better organized. The job of a CNS can become a real time-management nightmare. Poor time planning by CNSs is perhaps one of the worst problems in practice. It is a source of stress, a never-ending battle of trying to catch up. The worse your time management and planning skills are, the further behind you can fall.

It is very easy to become overwhelmed when you think of all of the things that need to be done. When considering things that should be dealt with, think about what must be done immediately, what needs to be done in the near future, and what can be put into the timeline of things to do. Make a list. If you have difficulty sorting out what needs to be completed by when, think about the tasks from a chi square perspective: high importance, low importance, urgent, nonurgent. A visual is an asset to most people—calendars, timelines, color-coded notes. Use any method that helps you sort and prioritize—paper check lists, reminder lists on the computer, a calendar app on your cellphone. Time management is only as good as your ability to stick to it.

LIFE/WORK BALANCE

With all of the new opportunities and challenges, a new CNS can be tempted to work long hours, but long days can leave you exhausted and can ultimately undermine your ability to achieve. Long hours at work can strain personal relationships, cause loss of enjoyable activities, and create additional stress both at home and at work.

A new CNS is particularly vulnerable to diving into more and more work and losing balance. Use time management strategies and goal setting to leave work at work when you walk out the door. Maintain the things in life that bring you pleasure. Set personal priorities to avoid being consumed by work. Do not lose your identity so much that the center of your being is focused on your CNS role.

Personal and professional priorities should be balanced to avoid feeling overwhelmed. Make "balance in all things" your mantra. Make a list of your priorities. Post the list in your office within view. When you are tempted to take on an additional project, read it, remember why you made this list, and ask, "Is this value added to my patient population, the staff, the system that supports the staff, and to me professionally? What else is on my plate? Can it wait? Can other projects be put on hold? Does it conflict with my personal goals?" (Covey, 1989, p. 106).

TIPPING POINT

The tasks and projects can be overwhelming. Patient care takes priority and can change your calendar in a moment. Meetings can take up much of your time. In the novice phase, if you have more than three to four meetings a week, you've probably gone too far. If these meetings take time away from focusing on the patients and staff, again, you have lost the battle with time management. You will have reached the tipping point—the "moment of critical mass, the threshold, the boiling point" (Gladwell, 2000, p. 12). Make appointments with yourself to revise your priorities, revisit timelines, negotiate duties. Reorganize, reprioritize, and reenergize.

LESSONS LEARNED

Let's examine the tale of two CNSs. The first CNS manages her time by outlining projects, addressing quantity of work, and making appointments for self time—time to think and work alone. She is able to keep current with research, is known for bringing evidence to the bedside, and has excellent outcomes within the three spheres. She meets her outbound train on time every day and does not take work home. She maintains her interests and relationships.

The second CNS is in her first CNS job. She was pleased and honored when asked to be involved in things. She makes patient care a priority even though her assigned units of coverage have grown from one to nine. She takes on most everything requested by staff in her units and is involved in multiple committees that all impact patient care in her specialty. She feels it is her responsibility to be the voice for nursing in the specialty area. She has no mentors.

She is known for being late and turning in work late—which is quite different from graduate school where she was envied by other students for being well prepared for class and never handing in an assignment late. She works 10- to 12-hour days and regularly takes work home. Her friends complain they never see her and stop inviting her to parties and events. She thinks that she has learned a lot and been a successful CNS.

The novice CNS was myself. A year after changing jobs, I was chatting with a staff nurse in one of the units I covered, and when I mentioned that I often thought of the nurses in that unit, she replied, "I don't know why, you were never there." Ouch!! Lesson learned. It took a life-changing experience to make me see that I was overwhelmed and was achieving little. I learned to balance my life and work—to be more like the first CNS example and less like the second.

Although I am tempted to overcommit, I have gotten better about asking for information before jumping in. I inquire about estimated time needed for the project, extent of the project, and possible benefits for patients and staff in my areas of responsibility. I look at what else is on my plate. I go through my calendar and see how much time I am spending out of my clinical area. If the project is more than I can afford to do, I go back to what my priorities are. I use the list method, with due dates, and committee responsibilities. I try to keep current with tasks and deadlines.

I have been involved in the Critical Care Committee (CCC) since I began my "new" job 10 years ago. About 5 years ago, I was appointed to be the first nurse cochair of the committee. There is enormous responsibility and practice throughout our facility through the work of the CCC. Prior to changing to a prioritization style of work, I put the agenda together, took the minutes and typed them, and implemented all the organizational-level practice changes within critical care. Because of this cochair position, I was constantly asked to do more and more with critical care and related issues. I always said yes. My life-changing experience helped me to change my approach to the CCC. I created cochairs and requested that they take over the agenda, the minutes, and make appropriate follow-ups to achieve project completion. I still work on projects for the CCC but no longer carry the full burden. The workload of this committee is much more balanced now.

I am more willing to refer individuals to my other CNS colleagues with expertise in the problem being presented. I no longer volunteer to take on everything. I elicit the help of my manager in looking at my commitments and offers of projects. As a result, I usually work about 9 hours a day. I leave on time and feel guilt free to do personal things. I enjoy spending my time sailing, meeting with friends, and traveling. I take vacations! I have finally realized that I am not indispensable. I understand that highly successful people say no all the time, and that successful people view the decision to say no as equally acceptable as the decision to say yes.

SUMMARY

The shortest full sentence in the English language is: "No." Remember it, as it will serve you well.

REFERENCES

Covey, S. R. (1989). *The seven habits of highly effective people; Restoring the character ethic.* New York, NY: Simon and Schuster.

Gladwell, M. (2000). *The tipping point* (p. 12). Boston, MA: Little, Brown, and Company. Retrieved from http://en.wikipedia.org/Time_management

CHAPTER 8

Finding a Mentor

VIVIAN DONAHUE

A wise man learns by the experiences of others.
A fool learns by nobody's experience.
An ordinary man learns by his own experience.

—Anonymous

After reading the chapter title, your first thought might be "Why do I need a mentor?" Mentoring has been suggested as a strategy for developing expertise and leadership in a mentee (McKinley, 2004) and for addressing horizontal violence and workplace bullying through role socialization and establishing a supportive environment (Echevarria, 2013; Frederick, 2014). A common thread in the literature describing mentorships includes professional development and social support. Given the complexity of the current state of health care, one might argue that successful assimilation into the clinical nurse specialist (CNS) role would be challenging without the support of a mentor(s). The question is not really *why* but *who* and *how many*? Before you embark on your journey to find a mentor, you must first consider: What is the value of a mentor? What are you hoping to achieve with this relationship?

The term *mentor* was first introduced in Homer's *Odyssey*. It has long been established in the business world but appears to have first entered the nursing literature in the late 1970s through the early research efforts on leadership by Connie Vance (1977). One of her research questions focused on whether national nursing leaders engaged in mentoring. Her findings revealed that the vast majority of those interviewed (93%) were actively mentoring others for future leadership roles and that they attributed much of their own success to their previous mentor relationships over the years (Nickitas, 2014).

Recognition of the benefits of mentoring for the professional development of registered nurses and advanced practice nurses is clearly established in the literature (Babcock, Rosebrock, & Snow, 2014; Gawlinski & Miller, 2011; Miga, Rauen, & Srsic-Stoehr, 2009).

The American Nurses Association (ANA) proposes mentoring as a means of supporting the advancement of practice, professionalism, and the overall quality of health care (ANA, 2010). In addition, the ANA states that nurses have an obligation to mentor colleagues and treat colleagues with respect, trust, and dignity (ANA, 2010). Magnet organizations have suggested that mentoring supports nurse retention by increasing satisfaction. Finally, the Institute of Medicine's (2010) *The Future of Nursing* report recommends that work organizations and professional organizations provide mentoring programs. Given the significant contributions and authenticity of each of these organizations, it becomes apparent that support exists for a mentoring experience and a positive experience can prove beneficial to all involved.

MENTOR AND MENTORING RELATIONSHIPS

There are numerous definitions for the terms "mentor" and "mentoring," each somewhat unique as the concept of mentoring continues to evolve. Definitions often include characteristics of the mentor, the mentee, and/or the mentoring relationship. They may also include expectations related to the mentoring relationship.

Mentors have been described as coaches, advisors, teachers, and friends and are often those individuals who possess qualities that others admire and strive to achieve (Kanaskie, 2006). A mentor is typically a trusted advisor, a teacher, and a person of wisdom (McKinley, 2004) who guides and develops a novice (Zerzan, Hess, Schur, Phillips, & Rigotti, 2009). Characteristics of good mentors include patience, enthusiasm, knowledge (Kanaskie, 2006), positive role modeling, a commitment to the mentoring relationship, a positive attitude, and a willingness to self-reflect in order to ensure a positive experience for mentees (Echevarria, 2013; Frederick, 2014). Vance proposes a unique characteristic of successful mentoring relationships, a concept she calls the "mentor intelligence" or MQ (Nickitas, 2014). The MQ comprises three elements: mentoring mentality (the knowing or knowledge required for the study, reflection, and practice of mentoring), the mentoring lens (the seeing aspect or viewing self and others as needing the relationship), and the mentoring momentum (actively creating and doing of it; Nickitas, 2014).

The term *preceptor* is often used interchangeably with mentor although there are distinctions. The term preceptor implies a short-term relationship, often assigned formally for educational purposes, and frequently involved in the evaluative process. The term mentor implies a long-term relationship, most often informally initiated, based on the mentee's needs. There are multiple stages that may be experienced throughout the relationship. Throughout the process, mentoring emphasizes advancing the mentee's professional goals, developing leadership skills, and opening doors to new growth opportunities (Hadidi, Lindquist, & Buckwalter, 2013). The relationship is ongoing and fluid and has significance as long as a mutual need exists between the mentor and mentee.

As there are individual characteristics descriptive of a positive mentor, there are also characteristics that would not promote an effective mentor–mentee relationship. Individuals who lack knowledge in communication skills and listening would not be effective mentors. A mentor must recognize that he or she is a role model and teacher. As such, the mentor must be able to advocate for the mentee and promote a positive learning experience.

Individuals who lack a positive outlook may not be able to provide this experience. Darling (1985) describes toxic mentors and suggests they fall into four categories: avoiders, dumpers, blockers, and destroyers or criticizers. We have all encountered individuals who exhibit one or more of these characteristics. Individuals who exhibit such behaviors would be excluded as ideal mentors.

This early work ties in with current work recognizing the toxic effects of bullying in the work place. Bullying behavior has been described as "verbal abuse, offensive conduct/behaviors that are threatening, humiliating or intimidating and work interference or sabotage that prevents work from being done" (Frederick, 2014, p. 588). Mentoring is a means of promoting professional satisfaction and supporting a work environment that provides zero tolerance for bullying behaviors.

In conjunction with mentor characteristics, there are techniques both formal and informal utilized by the most effective mentors to develop and support mentees in their professional growth. Frederick (2014) suggests techniques such as reflection, establishing expectations, and an awareness of the need for reciprocity to ensure professional gain and satisfaction for both the mentee and mentor. Additionally, three communication techniques that can be used by a mentor to build a supportive mentor–mentee relationship include questioning, thinking aloud, and debriefing (Frederick, 2014).

Mentoring is often used interchangeably with the terms *teaching, coaching, role modeling*, and *precepting*. Vance describes mentoring as a relationship that is essential for developing talent and facilitating professional success (Nickitas, 2014). She defines it as a developmental, empowering, nurturing relationship extending over time, in which mutual sharing, learning, and growth occur (Nickitas, 2014). "Mentoring promotes talent, achievement, leadership, knowledge, and skill development in a career" (p. 66). Role modeling, coaching, and teaching are all tools that can be utilized by a mentor to promote professional development and socialization of the mentee. Each of these tools plays a role in the mentoring process but alone is not sufficient in describing a mentor. "We are all role models, whether we like it or not. Our actions, words, body language, and behavior are always being observed by others" (Girard, 2006, p. 13). All mentors are role models, but not all role models are capable of mentoring.

An alternative description could include those characteristics that support a successful mentor–mentee relationship. Characterized as a powerful relationship between a novice and an expert, mentoring facilitates role socialization, creates a supportive environment, closes the gap between didactic and real-world experience, and promotes role success of the novice (Hill & Sawatzky, 2011).

Many factors affect one's ability to develop a mentoring relationship including gender, age, socioeconomic status, and personality (Roemer, 2002). Many of these factors continue to be of ongoing interest to researchers.

The literature is varied in its interpretation of these factors, suggesting that further research is needed to identify their impact on the mentor and mentee relationship.

The mentee also plays an active role in the mentoring relationship through demonstrating skills of self-assessment and by being receptive, open, and responsive to feedback and ideas (Zerzan et al., 2009). Managing up is a successful technique commonly used in the business world that has been shown to lead to a mutually satisfying relationship. The idea is that the mentee takes ownership of the relationship by establishing meeting agendas, asking questions, requesting feedback, and letting the mentor know what he or she needs (Zerzan et al., 2009). In seeking a mentor, the mentee must also identify those characteristics within that individual that will meet the mentee's professional needs. The mentee must identify a mentor with whom he or she is capable of sustaining a long-term relationship. Ideally a mentee should reflect on and identify personal strengths, weaknesses, and needs prior to seeking out a mentor.

PROFESSIONAL GROWTH

As with all developmental roles within the nursing profession, this relationship can be based on the principles of Patricia Benner's (2001) "novice-to-expert" approach. In this scenario, the mentor would be practicing at the expert level, and the mentee would be in the role of a novice. Role development would continue until a mutually agreed upon level of practice had been achieved. The relationship may become a lifetime commitment.

The characteristics most often ascribed to mentors help create an environment conducive to developing a long-term relationship. Patience is needed to provide an opportunity to the mentee to learn. Support and guidance are offered to help the mentee learn new tasks and to create an environment of success. Enthusiasm encourages the mentee to seek out new experiences and to avoid complacency (Fawcett, 2002). Knowledge is shared between the mentor and the mentee. Knowing his or her weaknesses allows the mentor to seek advice from experts and gain insight from the mentoring experience.

Mentoring involves mutual respect and reflection. Both mentor and mentee must be able to reflect objectively on their practice. This is a synergistic relationship meant to promote professional development for both the mentee and the mentor.

Mentoring impacts the mentor, the mentee, and the organization. "On a professional level, the mentor fosters pride for the nursing profession and contributes to the retention of a new nurse" (Patten, 2012, p. 18). Positive outcomes of the mentoring experience include improved retention and promoting professionalism.

Mentoring provides a unique opportunity for the CNS as both a mentor and a mentee. CNS students and new CNSs benefit from the clinical coaching and the mentoring relationship of an experienced CNS who can create a collegial environment for learning and build self-confidence in the role (France, 2006).

Role socialization has been clearly identified as an integral component of retention. Mentoring provides an opportunity to support colleagues and promote socialization. In terms of definitions alone we speak of identifying unit and organizational idiosyncrasies and assisting the mentee in gaining an understanding of these idiosyncrasies. This understanding promotes socialization and ultimately self-confidence in the new CNS.

An individual may choose to identify with one individual as a mentor or several individuals throughout his or her career. This process may evolve as the CNS develops. At varying times throughout a CNS's career, mentoring needs may need to be reassessed. Professional growth continues throughout a CNS's career and new opportunities present themselves. A mentor may or may not be someone within the role of CNS. The role of a CNS is expansive; the behavior or skill the CNS chooses to emulate may be found in other nursing leadership roles.

BENEFIT OF A MENTOR

Now that we have identified the characteristics of a mentor, it may be helpful to identify why one would choose to seek out a mentor. First we examine it from the perspective of the mentee. Feeling anxious and unsure of oneself is a natural sensation when undertaking a new endeavor. There are many benefits for the mentee once a mentor–mentee relationship has developed. One benefit is the process of becoming embedded within the organization. This process is facilitated through socialization, guidance in practice, and reassurances offered by the mentor. Each of these gains in turn promotes commitment to the organization and the profession. A process of enculturation develops and the mentee begins to grow and develop until he or she too becomes a mentor.

Mentoring relationships help both the mentor and the mentee develop a better understanding of each other's values and practices. Generational differences often create challenges to understanding each other's values. Developing a trusting relationship allows the participants to communicate in such a way that they begin to understand each other's belief systems and values.

A mentee is less likely to experience burnout and bullying and is more likely to feel rewarded in his or her career. A mentee is also more likely to become a mentor as he or she matures in the career, thereby creating a positive cycle within the profession. And finally, a mentee is more likely to advance in a professional career.

A mentor also benefits from this relationship. The mentor develops a better understanding of values and practices via the relationship with the mentee. Mentoring promotes growth and further practice development of the mentor. Some suggest that as the mentee becomes less dependent on the mentor, a more collegial relationship develops, creating a mutually supportive relationship.

There are also organizational benefits to mentoring. Retention is improved. Professional commitment on behalf of the organization becomes apparent. The organizational support for professional practice promotes an environment that encourages teamwork. A positive, healthy work environment ensues.

Mentoring promotes an understanding of the mission and vision of an organization through examination and discussion of the organization's values (McKinley, 2004).

Mentoring is a means to promote the profession of nursing. Mentoring helps develop future leaders within an organization and the profession (Kanaskie, 2006). "Nursing exists in a very complex world. To successfully navigate in that world, nurses need to mentor each other. Without mentoring, nurses become burned out and lose the spark of commitment to the profession" (Scott, 2005, p. 52). Many authors suggest that informal mentoring (those relationships that develop due to a shared or common interest) occurs frequently and spontaneously in nursing. It is this kind of ongoing commitment to the profession that will move nursing forward into the future.

COLLEGIAL AND ORGANIZATIONAL SUPPORT

Mentoring provides a structure for growth, professional satisfaction, and the ability to give back to colleagues and the profession. Mentoring can come in many forms. My first mentor was the nurse manager on the unit where I began my career. She was an incredibly intelligent, insightful, and giving nurse. Her commitment to the staff and the nursing profession was evident in every aspect of her practice. Nurse S. provided positive reinforcement to promote my strengths, helped me identify those areas for potential improvement, and recognized professional commitment in my practice. Nurse S. guided me toward a clinical recognition program to develop my practice and foster my self-confidence. She encouraged me to identify and speak about my career goals. When she discovered I had an interest in critical care nursing, she recommended me to her colleague who was the nurse manager of the medical intensive care unit. Without her encouragement and support, I would not have become a critical care CNS with more than 34 years of critical care experience.

Nurse S. was the first mentor in my career, but throughout my career I have identified those individuals whose qualities I have valued most and have sought their expertise and guidance. At every stage of my career, my needs have varied. While pursuing my master's degree in nursing, I had the opportunity to experience the role with CNSs in varied settings. I was also fortunate to be able to practice in my role as a CNS in an organization that supports the role. There are in excess of 50 CNSs in the organization, and all seek the guidance of colleagues in multiple roles, as each has a unique area of expertise. I have also had the opportunity to mentor amazing professionals who will soon be leaders in the profession. These opportunities have provided a great sense of professional growth and satisfaction to me. In my current role as a nursing director of a cardiac surgical intensive care unit and a cardiac intensive care unit in an academic medical center, I rely heavily on past and present mentors, many of whom are CNS colleagues.

SUMMARY

This journey began with the identification of two concepts in need of clarification. The first was the need to clearly articulate a definition of the term *mentor*. The second concept involved creating an understanding of the mentor–mentee relationship. Several definitions were offered, all with common denominators. Characteristics of a mentor were identified. The mutually beneficial relationship of mentor–mentee was explored. And finally, the benefits incurred by the mentee, the mentor, and the organization itself were discussed.

We are finally prepared to discuss how to find a mentor. Perhaps an algorithmic approach might be best (Figure 8.1). First, the mentee must reflect on his or her practice. Second, consideration must be given to which skills or practice abilities the mentee would like to emulate. An individual with similar values, goals, and practice must be willing to engage in and commit to the mentor–mentee relationship. And finally, a mutually rewarding, long-lasting relationship must develop between the two individuals. If this can be accomplished, one will have successfully found a mentor. This process is bidirectional and fluid and, as such, becomes a long-term or lifetime commitment.

In conclusion, mentoring promotes potential growth in the mentee and the mentor, and offers benefits to the organization. As evidenced by the age of the citations (ranging from the 1970s through 2015), mentoring is grounded in a solid foundation and continues to evolve. The complexity of health care and the rapidly growing expectations for the delivery of high-quality, safe patient care

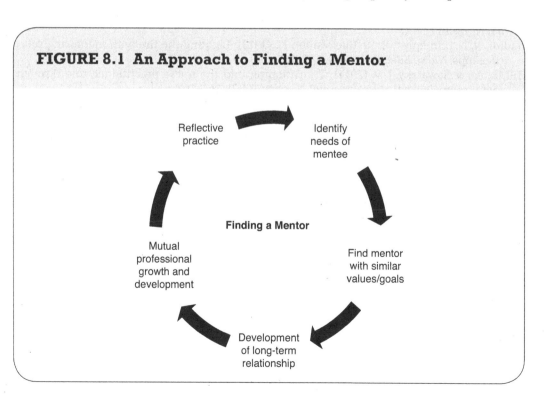

FIGURE 8.1 An Approach to Finding a Mentor

Reflective practice

Identify needs of mentee

Finding a Mentor

Find mentor with similar values/goals

Mutual professional growth and development

Development of long-term relationship

demand the expertise and leadership of nurses that can be developed through mentoring. A commitment must be made to the process by all involved for mentoring to be successful. Once committed to the process, the benefits appreciated by the mentee, the mentor, and the organization can be substantial.

REFERENCES

American Nurses Association. (2010). *Nursing: Scope and standards of practice* (2nd ed.). Silver Spring, MD: Author.

Babcock, P., Rosebrock, R., & Snow, B. (2014). Tips for mentoring advanced practice nursing students. *AACN Advances in Critical Care, 25*(4), 322–325.

Benner, P. (2001). *From novice to expert: Excellence and power in clinical nursing practice.* Menlo Park, CA: Addison-Wesley.

Darling, L. A. (1985). What to do about toxic mentors. *Journal of Nursing Administration, 15*(5), 43–44.

Echevarria, I. M. (2013). Change your appetite: Stop "eating the young" and start mentoring. *Nursing Critical Care, 8*(3), 21–14.

Fawcett, D. L. (2002). Mentoring: What it is and how to make it work (Research/Education). *Association of Operating Room Nurses, 75*(5), 950–954.

France, N. E. M. (2006). Socializing clinical nurse specialist students for practice. *Clinical Nurse Specialist, 20*(2), 97–99.

Frederick, D. (2014). Bullying, mentoring, and patient care. *Association of Operating Room Nurses, 99*(5), 587–593.

Gawlinski, A. & Miller, P. (2011). Advancing nursing research through a mentorship program for nurses. *AACN Advances in Critical Care, 22*(3), 190–200.

Girard, N. J. (2006). Like it or not you are a role model. *Association of Operating Room Nurses, 84*(1), 13–15.

Hadidi, N. N., Lindquist, R., & Buckwalter, K. (2013). Lighting the fire with mentoring relationships. *Nurse Educator, 38*(4), 157–163.

Hill, L. A., & Sawatzky, J. V. (2011). Transitioning into the nurse practitioner role through mentorship. *Journal of Professional Nursing, 27*(3), 161–167.

Institute of Medicine. (2010). *The future of nursing: Leading change, advancing health.* Washington, DC: National Academies Press.

Kanaskie, M. L. (2006). Mentoring: A staff retention tool. *Critical Care Nursing Quarterly, 29*(3), 248–252.

McKinley, M. G. (2004). Mentoring matters: Creating, connecting, empowering. *AACN Clinical Issues, 15*(2), 205–214.

Miga, K.C., Rauen, C., & Srsic-Stoehr, K. (2009). Strategies for success: Orienting to the role of a clinical nurse specialist in critical care. *AACN Advances in Critical Care, 20*(1), 47–54.

Nickitas, D. (2014) Mentorship in nursing: An interview with Connie Vance. *Nursing Economics, 32*(2), 65–69.

Patten, C. S. (2012). Mentor and protege: A mutually beneficial relationship. *Lippincott's Career Directory,* 17–18.

Roemer, L. (2002). Women CEOs in health care: Did they have mentors? *Health Care Management Review, 27*(4), 57–67.

Scott, E. S. (2005). Peer-to-peer mentoring: Teaching collegiality. *Nurse Educator, 30*(2), 52–56.

Vance, C. N. (1977). *A group profile of contemporary influentials in American nursing.* Doctoral dissertation. Teachers College, Columbia University, New York, NY.

Zerzan, J. T., Hess, R., Schur, E., Phillips, R., & Rigotti, N. (2009). Making the most of mentors: A guide for mentees. *Academic Medicine, 84*(1), 140–144.

CHAPTER 9

Using the Internet: Guide to Internet-Based Resources

BARBARA MANZ FRIESTH
SUSAN K. B. JONES

The landmark Institute of Medicine (IOM, 2010) report on the future of nursing made several recommendations for improving health. Key among them was the recommendation to ensure that nurses be engaged in lifelong learning. Internet-based resources reduce the burden for access to lifelong learning resources, but being aware of and using the plethora of resources available is essential to clinical nurse specialist (CNS) practice. Staying abreast of the changing information requires CNSs to remain current on changing practice trends for the populations of patients with whom they work. This means that CNSs must stay connected to all of the sources of information that have the potential to impact their practice, their patients, and the organizations with which they work.

Staying connected includes using the technology and the Internet. CNSs use the Internet to remain connected to professional organizations, to search and find the best evidence that influences the way care is provided to patients and families, and to stay connected to national and international organizations conducting research and setting standards of practice for their patient populations. The importance of professional organizations and networking is addressed later in this toolkit. The focus of this section is the multiple ways that a CNS can use Internet resources to provide and support quality patient care.

Although these resources could be organized in a variety of ways, for the purposes of this chapter they will be organized by:

- Global resources as they relate to evidence-based practice
- Resources that influence organizational decisions
- Specialty patient population resources and newer technologies allowing point of care access and networking

By no means should this be considered an exhaustive list of resources, but it should provide a beginning framework of the types of resources available for you and the professionals and patients with whom you work.

ORGANIZATIONAL RESOURCES

Irrespective of the CNS's population specialty, national groups influence the care of those patients. Figure 9.1 (Gelinas, 2007) represents some of the national policy-making groups and specialty organizations that influence the way care is provided. It is incumbent upon CNSs to be aware of recommendations that are promoted by these organizations. Although it is beyond the scope of this text to include all of the electronic addresses for these organizations, a simple electronic search for these organizations will provide the appropriate addresses. A brief examination of each of these sites will assist in identifying tools prepared to support the work of each group. For example, information found on the Institute for Healthcare Improvement (2015) website (ihi.org) includes information about the science of improvement within health

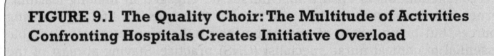

FIGURE 9.1 The Quality Choir: The Multitude of Activities Confronting Hospitals Creates Initiative Overload

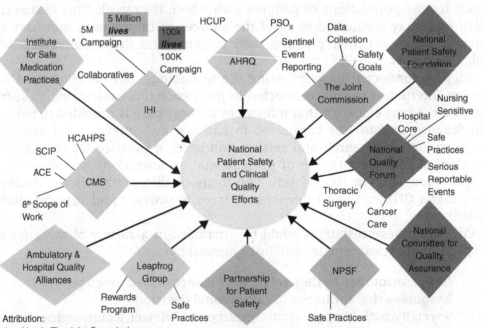

Attribution:
Jerod Loeb, The Joint Commission
ACE, achieving customer excellence; CMS, Centers for Medicare & Medicaid Services; HCAHPS, Hospital Consumer Assessment of Health Care Providers and Systems; HCUP, Health Care Cost and Utilization Project; IHI, Institute for Healthcare Improvement; NPSF, National Patient Safety Foundation; PSO, Patient Safety Organization; SCIP, Surgical Care Improvement Project.

From Lillie S. Gelinas, RN, BSN, MSN, FAAN, system vice president and chief nursing officer at CHRISTUS Health. Reprinted with permission.

care systems. Contained within this website are tools and resources to assist health care professionals with quality improvement knowledge and skills. Similar resources focused in their respective areas can be found by accessing any of these organizations online, and is helpful in providing the background on national initiatives in an easy-to-use format.

EVIDENCE-BASED PRACTICE RESOURCES

Resources for finding the evidence on which to base practice are slowly becoming more accessible through open access requirements and Internet resources. Despite some increased accessibility, staying abreast of the ever-changing research base upon which CNSs base practice decisions can be a full-time job. To remain successful in this arena, it is important to maximize your efforts. This means knowing the most helpful Internet sites, identifying which (if any) databases you have access to through your organization or school, and developing a close working relationship with the librarians in both locations. In order to understand where to begin to look, it is important to understand the many different types of information available for review. Where to look for information will be determined by the type of information needed. For individual primary research articles, begin by searching a scientific publication database such as PubMed (searches MEDLINE) or CINHAL. Electronic access to PubMed (pubmed.gov) is available through the National Library of Medicine and the National Institutes of Health without subscription; access to the citation and the abstract for those articles is available at no charge. However, to access many of the full-text versions of the articles, users must either purchase the article directly from PubMed or have access through a subscription. In order to search the CINHAL database, a subscription to a service is required; EBSCO is the current owner of the CINAHL database. Many hospitals have subscriptions to services that enable online searching and retrieval of research articles. If your organization does not have a subscription of this type, consider contacting a librarian at a local, publicly funded university and explore developing a relationship. Explore what the librarian might be able to do to help you access the databases to which the institution subscribes. In addition, Google Scholar (scholar.google.com) provides a free option for searching broadly among scholarly literature, with links to sources that may require payment for full access.

While these types of databases are helpful in finding primary research articles, many of the topics that are important to CNS practice have been broadly researched and may have variable or conflicting findings. When systematic reviews of the literature are available, the information helps ensure that practice decisions are made using the best information available, and decisions are not necessarily based on a single study. Helpful sites for determining whether a systematic review of the literature has been performed include sites from the Cochrane Library, the Joanna Briggs Institute (JBI), and others found in Table 9.1. The Cochrane Library performs systematic reviews of research related to health care and health policy, specifically related to making informed

TABLE 9.1 Useful Websites for Clinical Nurse Specialists

Website	URL
PubMed	pubmed.gov
Cochrane Library	cochranelibrary.com
Joanna Briggs Institute (JBI)	connect.jbiconnectplus.org
Agency for Healthcare Research and Quality (AHRQ)	www.ahrq.gov
Centers for Disease Control and Prevention (CDC)	www.cdc.gov
National Guidelines Clearinghouse (NGC)	www.guideline.gov
National Quality Measures Clearinghouse (NQMC)	www.qualitymeasures.ahrq.gov
Registered Nurses Association of Ontario (RNAO)—Nursing Best Practice Guidelines	rnao.ca/bpg
American Association of Critical-Care Nurses—Clinical Practice	www.aacn.org
Oncology Nurses Society—Practice Resources	www.ons.org/practice-resources
Hartford Institute for Geriatric Nursing	www.hartfordign.org
Society of Critical Care Medicine	www.sccm.org

choices about interventions. Access to the Cochrane Library is available in the United States by subscription only (Cochrane Library, 2015). Check with your organization and/or your higher education libraries to determine whether you have access to this information.

The JBI website provides information based on systematic reviews of the literature as well, but these reviews go beyond reviews of effectiveness. The JBI site also provides reviews of studies based upon the feasibility, appropriateness, and meaningfulness of health care practices (Joanna Briggs Institute [JBI], 2015). Information from the JBI systematic reviews of the literature (SRL) is available in several formats; the two most popular are the SRLs and the Best Practice Information Sheets (BPIS). The full-text SRL provides detailed information including the search strategy and in-depth information about the articles themselves. The BPISs provide a synopsis of the information from the SRL in an easy-to-read format. Additionally, the BPISs contain recommendations for practice as well as suggestions for future research. Access to the complete systematic reviews is available through membership only; access to many of the BPISs on JBI is available without subscription through the JBI website.

Beyond being aware of and being able to find systematic reviews of the literature, CNSs use the Internet to locate and learn about national and international guidelines for care. These clinical practice guidelines come from a variety of organizations and in several differing formats. Table 9.1 lists web addresses that may be helpful in identifying clinical practice guidelines for different populations. Each site has a search option that may be helpful in narrowing the scope of interest.

SPECIALTY RESOURCES

Specialty organizations have become increasingly influential in setting the standards for providing patient care. Some organizations provide free access to the information related to their specialty populations, while others require membership for access. This membership requirement is another reason involvement in a specialty organization can be very beneficial to the CNS. Table 9.1 includes some of the specialty organization websites that allow nonmember access to the best-practice information impacting particular populations of interest. Organizations such as the Infusion Nursing Society and the Association of peri-Operative Registered Nurses have a plethora of information that is available through membership. (Please do not be offended if your specialty organization is not included. As stated previously, many organizations require membership in order to access their resource information. Those websites were not included.)

HANDHELD TECHNOLOGY

Increasingly resource information is also accessible via handheld technology, including either specialized apps or websites that are optimized for viewing on smartphones or tablets. For example, the Cochrane Library has an app for tablets that includes full text as well as integrated videos and podcasts associated with the reviews. PubMed also has an app for searching and reviewing literature that is compatible with handheld devices. In addition, many of the organizational websites previously mentioned are designed to be viewed in mobile-friendly formats, and have been optimized for use on handheld devices. The number of apps available for specific resources is increasing rapidly, so a quick search for the specific site/organization you are interested in will yield the timeliest information.

SOCIAL MEDIA AND DISCUSSION FORUMS

While adhering to best practices for use of social media (National Council of State Boards of Nursing [NCSBN], 2015), it is important to note that some tools in social media are finding a significant role in health care. Twitter is a microblogging platform meant to share real-time, short bursts of information of about 140 characters or less, called "tweets." Twitter is increasingly being used at professional conferences using "hashtags" or the "#" symbol to identify easily searchable bits of information on a given topic or event. In addition, many of the organizations and resources previously mentioned have twitter feeds that CNSs can follow to receive up-to-date information on new and trending topics, with links to more in-depth information than is available on the Twitter platform.

Most of the specialty organizations have discussion forums within their websites that allow members to exchange ideas and receive feedback on posted issues. This type of networking provides an archived record of conversations, which benefit users within their own time demands not requiring real-time simultaneous communication.

And finally, LinkedIn is a professional social network that allows users to connect with others based on professional interests. Members of LinkedIn create a user profile that identifies them by profession and specialty, and allows users to seek out similar profiles. It can be an excellent network to find other CNSs interested in like-minded issues or topics, and is particularly helpful in breaking down geographic hurdles in networking.

LISTSERVS

Listservs were created as web-based discussion forums. Subscribers of a listserv form a network with others of similar interests. Members can ask and respond to questions, thus gaining advice, perspective, or support about shared concerns. The National Association of Clinical Nurse Specialists Listserv (NACNS-list-owner@mail-list.com) is a popular listserv for CNSs regardless of specialty. Other listservs of interest to CNSs are advanced nursing practice (ANPACC@ yahoogroups.com) and pediatric advanced practice nursing (PICUAPN@ yahoogroups.com) sites.

Listservs gained popularity in the late 1990s as Internet access expanded. However, with advances in social media, listservs are being replaced by some of the options discussed in the previous section.

The information included in this chapter is representative of information available to CNSs and the organizations with whom they work, but it is by no means an exhaustive compilation. The information represents a framework on which CNSs can build to use the ever-changing content that is available via the Internet and technology to guide the care they and their organizations provide.

REFERENCES

Cochrane Library. (2015). *Access options for the Cochrane Library*. Retrieved from http://www.cochranelibrary.com/help/access-options-for-the-cochrane-library.html

Gelinas, L. S. (2007). *National nursing leadership update: A focus on nursing care and clinical quality*. Presented at VHA Oklahoma-Arkansas Joint CNO Meeting, September 21, 2007.

Institute for Healthcare Improvement. (2015). *Improving health and health care worldwide.* Retrieved from http://ihi.org/ihi

Institute of Medicine. (2010). *The future of nursing: Leading change, advancing health.* Retrieved from http://books.nap.edu/openbook.php?record_id=12956&page=R1

Joanna Briggs Institute. (2015). *About the Joanna Briggs Institute.* Retrieved from http://connect.jbiconnectplus.org/About.aspx

National Council of State Boards of Nursing. (2015). *Social media guidelines for nurses.* Retrieved from https://www.ncsbn.org/347.htm

PART III

GAINING MOMENTUM

CHAPTER 10

Leading Groups

MELISSA A. LOWDER

Sure, you've been a member of a committee before, but now you have been asked to chair a committee—to lead a group. Whether it's a new group or an existing one, who better than a clinical nurse specialist (CNS) to lead it? A core competency of CNS practice is to "lead nursing and multidisciplinary groups in implementing innovative patient care programs that address issues across the full continuum of care for different population groups and/or different specialties" (National Association of Clinical Nurse Specialists [NACNS], 2004, p. 36). CNSs have the education, experience, and clinical competency to lead groups for the purpose of patient care innovation or clinical program development, implementation, and evaluation.

TYPES OF GROUPS

What type of group will you lead? Most often, groups are a collection of individuals working toward the same purpose. They are developed to disseminate information, seek opinions, and/or solve problems (Huber, 2014). Based on the purpose of the group, it may be structured in the organization as a task group (task force), a standing committee, a subcommittee/ad hoc group, or a council.

A task group consists of several persons who work together to accomplish a specific time-limited assignment (Sullivan, 2013). Groups of nurses working together to write a new policy on restraint care or to design a patient educational program are examples of task groups. In this type of group, members work independent of administrative leadership. With task groups, a CNS may bring the group together, clarify the charge and timeline, ensure that members have all needed resources, and then allow them to work independently, serving only as a facilitator.

Committees are created to address specific ongoing issues and may be single discipline or multidisciplinary. Committees exist as structural elements in the organization and may be created by bylaws or administrative units. In health care settings, standing committees usually involve several service areas or disciplines (Sullivan, 2013). An example of a standing committee would be a patient safety committee that is responsible for monitoring and improving patient safety. Committees are very common in organizations and require strong leadership for efficient operations and targeted outcomes.

An ad hoc group or committee is designed to address a specific immediate need. Like a task force, it is a temporary group that functions within a specific time frame. Some ad hoc committees are formed as a subcommittee of a larger committee and charged with addressing one or two interrelated topics that are under the responsibility of a larger committee. For example, a subcommittee to address falls may be formed from the patient safety committee. This new group would be charged with a specific task that is under the goals and purpose of the larger group. Once the ad hoc committee has addressed the topic, the ad hoc group would disband. In this example, responsibility for ongoing monitoring of improved outcomes related to falls would return to the larger patient safety committee.

In health care, councils are typically groups with broad representation of a population with decision-making and oversight responsibilities. For example, on a local level, unit councils have representation of all the staff on an individual unit. Clinical practice councils and staff councils are examples of organization-wide groups that have representatives from all nursing departments. While CNSs may or may not be responsible for leading these groups, there is a leadership role that the CNS may fill to help these groups accomplish their goals.

CNSs also lead groups that do not include meetings and agendas, such as a multidisciplinary rounding team. In this situation many of the same principles of groups apply. A multidisciplinary rounding team still needs clear vision and purpose, defined membership, a predetermined schedule, and, above all, leadership.

CHARTERING YOUR GROUP

A charter is a way to organize a group so that the key elements are well defined and communicated. Start by asking, "What is the *purpose* of this group?" It is very important that the group you are leading be thoughtfully constructed and have clear direction. The group must also fit with the goals, vision, and mission of the organization, committee, or unit that it is intended to serve. The group's purpose may be delegated by an administrator or written into organizational bylaws. However, for situations in which a CNS identifies a need to develop a group to fill a distinct need, the purpose should be developed by its members within the group. Regardless of the reason for the group, it is essential that those who elect or are appointed to participate in the group know, understand, and agree upon the purpose of the group and the end product or *deliverables* expected.

Who should be the *members* of the group? CNSs bring leadership and clinical talent to a group; however, CNSs do not work in isolation. Collaboration and teamwork are essential to achieving high-quality outcomes and cost control in client care (Huber, 2014). A diverse group of professionals collectively possesses greater knowledge and information, increases the likelihood of acceptance and understanding of the decisions made by the group, and enhances cooperation in implementation of any plan or intervention (Sullivan, 2013).

When deciding who should be in the group, first determine any standing members or required members. For some committees, bylaws or accreditation guidelines may specify members—not the individual person, but the credentials of the person. For example, accreditation guidelines may specify that some committees include physician members, while other committees may specify interdisciplinary membership. In addition to determining the required members, assess the stakeholders associated with the group's purpose and expected outcome. Make sure all key stakeholders have a voice in the group. It is easy to have too many members in a group—groups between 10 and 12 individuals are the most efficient for a committee, although some councils can have up to 40 to 50 members (Roussel, 2013).Giving voice to all stakeholders without adding members requires some thoughtful consideration. It may be necessary to select only one person from a large stakeholder group and charge this person with communicating with key members of the larger group, or the group may decide to publish reports, hold informational meetings, or seek input and feedback from stakeholders in other ways. In the end, a CNS should help ensure that the group is not overpopulated, does not include unnecessary members, and is not missing important key stakeholders.

Avoid the temptation to rely on established clinical leaders or administrators to participate in the group. As much as these members add strength to the group, it is essential that you include the "end users"—those persons who work with the targeted patient population and who will be responsible for implementing the outcomes of the group's work. For example, when organizing a group to evaluate and select products and supplies, those clinicians who will utilize the products and supplies should be included. Including direct caregivers may create some challenges in scheduling meetings; however, caregivers can provide vital information that helps shape the work of the team and leads to better acceptance during the implementation phase. Clearly communicating the group members' expectations, including time commitments, may help avoid poor attendance and/or lack of participation. Change the day or time that the group meets, if necessary, to motivate individuals who may be reluctant due to scheduling concerns. Give members clear assignments with timelines and benchmarks for accountability. CNSs are group leaders and should keep the group goals moving forward; avoid or promptly resolve individual issues that create obstacles in meeting goals and timelines.

At times, a CNS may need to invite ad hoc members to join the group for a short period of time. For example, when reviewing data to determine responses to emergency situations, if the group identifies telecommunications issues that are slowing response times, the group should ask a member of the telecommunications department to join the group to brainstorm and problem solve these specific issues. Once the issues are resolved, the ad hoc member may be excused. It is important to be respectful of everyone's time. It may be necessary for selected key individuals to be present for only part of a meeting, during which a particular agenda's items are addressed, or it may not be necessary for some members to attend every meeting. Let the agenda guide the attendance for each meeting.

Schedules need to be determined well ahead of time. The frequency of meeting should be determined by the nature and urgency of the work. For example, a multidisciplinary rounding team may need to assemble twice a week in order to accomplish patient care plan revisions, whereas a departmental committee with the primary purpose of approving policies may have to meet only every other month. The time of day at which your group meets should be carefully considered. Groups that have physician members tend to be better attended early in the morning. Scheduling meetings for groups that contain members who work various shifts can be challenging. Work with the unit manager to plan appropriately to allow for staff nurses to participate in group work.

The *agenda* of any meeting should be driven by the purpose for which the group was formed. Agendas should be distributed before the meeting (usually 1 week) in order to give members time to prepare and thoughtfully consider the items. Depending on the group's charter, members may be able to contribute to or amend the agenda. Items should be prioritized on the agenda to allow enough time to address all items on the list. Standing reports and recurring updates can be distributed with the agenda as written reports, thus maximizing group interactions during the meeting. For each item, indicate the time allotted and the person responsible for presenting or reporting on that topic. To relay the purpose of each agenda item, use decisive phrases such as "to recommend" or "to make a final decision" for those items for which action is expected, and "to discuss" or "to consider" for those for which the purpose is *not* to drive action (McConnell, 2014). In this way, the group members are given a clear message about what the expected outcome is for the topics included in the meeting.

DISCUSSION AND FOLLOW-UP

The scope, function, and authority of the group must be clearly stated (Liebler & McConnell, 2012). Is the purpose of the group to deliberate and make recommendations; does it have the authority to make decisions that are binding? If the purpose is to formulate recommendations, it must be clear to whom those recommendations are to be given. To whom is the group accountable? As the group leader, you are responsible for communicating the vision, strategy, and outcomes of your team to the person or group to whom the group is accountable.

Whatever group a CNS is leading, there must be a clear understanding of the group's decision-making authority. The group's authority will depend on the status of the members of the group, the nature of the decisions, and the impact of those decisions on the organization. If the group is not able to implement decisions independently, a CNS may need to secure an administrative sponsor. If the group's work involves expectations from physician colleagues, securing a physician champion is a wise move as well.

Groups may have a very formal process structure, or may be very informal. As with membership, the structure of the group may be determined by bylaws or accreditation guidelines or other influences. The final structure depends on the authority and charge of the group. For instance, a board of directors that has administrative and fiscal responsibility for an organization is a very structured group. There are required agenda items, and minutes must be taken, approved, and archived. Standing committees usually require minutes that include attendance, discussion topics, and decisions or actions that result from committee voting. Task groups and ad hoc groups may not need minutes; these groups may submit one final report to the primary committee or administrator.

DOCUMENTATION

It is good practice to document the work of every group. When minutes are required, it is very difficult for one person to both facilitate a meeting and take minutes, so a CNS should secure clerical support whenever possible. If this cannot be accomplished, ask for a volunteer from the group to take minutes. Keep in mind that the documentation of the proceedings may serve as the evidence that accreditation standards are being met. Therefore, minutes should be accurate, specific, detailed, and reflect all decisions and action plans with responsible persons assigned to them. Some key elements that should be contained in the minutes are as follows:

- Name of the group
- Date and location of the meeting
- Time the meeting started and adjourned
- Attendance: list those present as well as those who were absent (be sure to note absences as excused or not excused)
- Any guests or substitute members in attendance
- A statement that the previous minutes were approved
- Discussion topics and discussion leader
- A summary of the discussion and any subsequent decisions made—be sure to document the final decision that was made
- All actions to be taken, with responsible party and time frame in which the action should be completed
- Items to be continued onto the next meeting's agenda
- Date, place, and time of the next meeting

Minutes should be made available to members within a reasonable time frame and retained in accordance with your organization's document retention policy (usually between 3 and 5 years).

ENVIRONMENT AND SETUP

Ensure that the physical environment supports good group interaction. Make sure the temperature is acceptable and noise is kept to a minimum. Arranging seating in such a way that all members of the group can see one another often helps facilitate discussion and a feeling of equality among members. Classroom-type arrangements can suggest a lecturing environment, where one person dominates the discussion.

Because participants of meetings often work in multiple different buildings or off-site locations, gathering members in one location can present challenges. Although it is not ideal, consider substituting some face-to-face meetings with conference calls or allow some members from more distant sites to join by telephone or webinar. Consider the impact it may have on the group dynamics or meeting agenda before proceeding. Plan accordingly for those individuals who will be joining via phone or the web. Have a plan to ensure those individuals can view all presentations and handouts. Demonstrations are done best via a webinar. Documents can be stored in a share drive that all participants can access or have e-mailed prior to the meetings. Any handouts that are brought to the meeting without prior notification should be scanned or faxed to participants joining virtually. Keep in mind that meetings that include brainstorming or flowcharting processes are difficult to conduct using phone conference methods. When using phone conferencing technology, be sure to send any documents to the member(s) before the meeting.

SECURING RESOURCES

The formation of a work group is not without cost to the organization. Therefore, a group must be efficient in accomplishing its goals and meeting the overall purpose. As the leader, you are responsible for articulating the value and impact that a group has on your organization and for ensuring that the group produces outcomes that provide a return on the resource investment made. The leader should obtain the resources necessary to efficiently accomplish the work of the group. One important resource is clerical support to help with the operational elements of the group work. In addition to writing minutes, a clerical assistant can arrange for meeting space, prepare materials, and assist with communications with others.

Good group meetings can be enhanced by ensuring that the appropriate equipment and supplies are available. Easels and flip charts can be essential in documenting brainstorming sessions. Electronic equipment such as computers and LCD panels can enhance the effectiveness of group presentations. Plan ahead and have all necessary equipment and supplies available. Test electronic equipment prior to the meeting to avoid wasting time troubleshooting mechanical failures or replacing missing items.

LEADER RESPONSIBILITIES

The leader sets the tone of the meeting. Start and end meetings promptly. Starting late gives positive reinforcement to latecomers. Establish a clear expectation that meetings will start on time; members will quickly adjust their schedules to avoid being late. Most meetings typically last between 60 and 90 minutes. If the meeting is to exceed 90 minutes, time for a break should be allotted in the schedule.

Open meetings by concisely and clearly communicating an overview of the focus, task, or agenda for the meeting. During a meeting, summarize decisions and action items to bring clarity to discussions, to reinforce individual responsibility for action items, and to assist in accurately recording minutes. At the end of the meeting, read aloud a list of action items and the person responsible for each item.

Setting the milieu is also the responsibility of the group leader. Simple gestures such as thanking members for their attendance and recognizing individuals for their effort and contribution will facilitate a feeling of worth and appreciation among members. Expressions of appreciation will encourage quality performance and set a precedent for how all group members should interact with one another.

Soliciting ideas, opinions, and information prior to a meeting can be helpful. For example, if a CNS is facilitating a group responsible for product selection in a hospital, it may be valuable to send the proposed agenda and list of items up for discussion to members of the committee prior to the meeting so that they may research the necessity and use of the products and therefore best represent the needs of their unit during the meeting. This will also ensure that good, informed decisions are made and decision making is not delayed to a subsequent meeting. For all meetings, sending advance copies of documents for review should facilitate more thoughtful discussion; provide opportunity for members to validate concerns by checking existing guidelines, empiric evidence, or expert opinion; and thus make for more considered discussion at the meeting.

Some other responsibilities of the group leader are:

- Periodically review team progress and goal attainment
- Respond enthusiastically to all suggestions and ideas of group members
- Allow everyone in the group the opportunity to be heard
- Entertain various problem-solving methods and potential solutions
- Do not give your opinion until everyone else has spoken
- Keep track of the time and keep on schedule
- Assign tasks as needed
- Role-model and inspire others to continue their focus on the goals of the group
- Correlate group activities with the work of other related groups or departments
- Ensure compliance with mandated expectations and deadlines

Remember, groups that are productive tend to build on ideas of members by finding the strengths in a suggestion. In groups that are not productive, members spend time finding the weaknesses of an idea. A CNS can facilitate a productive group by asking members to build on ideas with statements like "What is good about that idea?" or "How can we strengthen that idea so it will work with our patients?" Keep the creative juices flowing by rewarding innovative thinking and minimizing devil's advocate–type arguments.

GROUP MEMBER RESPONSIBILITIES

For clinical staff nurses and salaried staff, being selected to serve as a group member should be viewed as an honor. Members possess the important knowledge and skills needed for a specific outcome. As group leaders, CNSs should communicate that being a member of a group is important and comes with responsibilities. Make sure the members of the group know the expectations and responsibilities of membership.

Attendance at group meetings is a clear expectation. Some absences are expected; however, members should review agenda items and send feedback or send a designated representative to a meeting when appropriate. In some situations, for attendance purposes a member who sends a designated representative may be considered an excused absence (in lieu of unexcused absence). Continued membership on a committee or work group may be dependent on attendance; after a specified number of unexcused absences (often three), the member is removed from the committee. The attendance requirement and consequences should be stated up front.

Group members should come to meetings prepared to participate. This means having obtained and/or read all pertinent materials ahead of time. For example, if a policy is to be approved during a meeting, time to read the policy will not be available during the meeting—the meeting will include discussion and voting on action items only. Members should also prepare by obtaining additional information to answer any questions, validate concerns, or identify alternatives. Being prepared to offer ideas that address problem areas will keep the work of the committee moving forward.

Group members should actively participate in discussions by offering feedback, suggestions, and ideas in a respectful and professional manner. This may be difficult for members new to communicating ideas in groups. When a committee includes inexperienced members, a CNS leader should be creative in assisting these members to contribute. Actively seeking ideas by calling upon individuals or using a round-robin approach to solicit input from the less verbal members of the group may be helpful in drawing out new members. It is equally important to control the talkers in the group so everyone has a chance to contribute.

Although the group leader is responsible for keeping meetings on track, it is also the responsibility of each group member to help the discussion stay on topic and to the point. It is not helpful for any member of the group (including the leader) to get sidetracked by tangents or "soap box" lectures. As the leader, avoid these nonconstructive behaviors and stop others by bringing them back to the initial topic. Some tangential conversations may actually be good agenda items for future meetings, so consider suggesting adding the topic to a future agenda.

As the leader, clearly communicate the expectation that members complete assigned action items/tasks. Group progress slows when assignments are not completed in a timely manner. If group members repeatedly fail to complete assignments, the leader must intervene. Confront member(s) in a private setting using a nonthreatening and caring manner. Give the member the opportunity to explain why the task was not completed. It could be that the member did not understand the task, did not have adequate resources, or was faced with unplanned or uncontrollable circumstances that prevented the work from being finished. Give the member an opportunity to reflect on why the task was not completed and to either renew his or her commitment to complete the task or hand it off with no repercussions. If the member demonstrates a pattern of completing work late or failing to complete work, the CNS should suggest that this may not be the best time for the person to serve on the committee/group. Resignation will facilitate appointment of a new member until such time as the person can devote more time and energy to the group.

Finally, where the group is charged with implementation, members should understand that it is an expectation that they assist with implementation of action plans. Members should become champions of the change and resources for implementation within their peer groups. Members should seek feedback about both the implementation process and the action plan itself. The group should also facilitate collecting and analyzing evaluation data and reporting.

MENTORING NEW GROUP LEADERS

Members of the group should be given opportunities to develop professionally, and CNSs can make good mentors. As you gain experience as a CNS group leader, try giving some members assignments that you typically would perform. For example, ask one or two group members to conduct a literature review or search for guidelines or standards. Facilitate members in developing skills. Teaching staff nurses to perform literature reviews may take more of your time initially but is well worth the investment. Another way to mentor the group members and build skills is to rotate meeting leaders. Rotating leaders will give members opportunity to develop skills in conducting a meeting. As you identify the various strengths of the members, begin matching strengths with opportunities. For example, a member skilled at leading meetings could be asked to coordinate an ad hoc group to address a specific problem.

REVISITING YOUR CHARTER

Groups should be subject to periodic review of purpose and function (Liebler & McConnell, 2012). This review may help to either acknowledge the importance of the group or provide redirection. In evaluating the group, ask:

- Do the proceedings and production of the group still fit with the purpose, goals, and mission that were originally outlined?
- Would the organization be affected if this group were eliminated?
- Do the day, time, and frequency of meetings meet with the needs of the members and organization?
- Is the group the right size and are the necessary stakeholders present?

If the answer to any of these questions is no, you may want to consider changes. Present the analysis to the group for discussion, and share findings with the person to whom the group is accountable.

I hope that this summary on leading groups was enjoyable and useful. The CNS is ideal for this role and can make an impact on an organization as both a formal and informal leader. It has been my pleasure to work with some phenomenal groups in some fantastic work in my organization. Good luck in all your endeavors!

REFERENCES

Huber, D. (2014). *Leadership and nursing care management* (5th ed.). St. Louis, MO: Elsevier Saunders.

Liebler, J. G., & McConnell, C. R. (2012). *Management principles for health professionals* (6th ed.). Sudbury, MA: Jones and Bartlett.

McConnell, C. R. (2014). *Umiker's management skills for the new health care supervisor* (6th ed.). Boston, MA: Jones and Bartlett.

National Association of Clinical Nurse Specialists (NACNS). (2004). *Statement on clinical nurse specialist practice and education* (2nd ed.). Harrisburg, PA: Author.

Roussel, L. (2013). *Management and leadership for nurse administrators* (6th ed.). Burlington, MA: Jones and Bartlett.

Sullivan, E. J. (2013). *Effective leadership and management in nursing* (8th ed.). Boston, MA: Pearson Education.

CHAPTER 11

Mentoring Staff

PATRICIA A. FOSTER

Clinical nurse specialists (CNSs) promote excellent patient care through the power of mentoring staff. Consider this mentoring experience: A large telemetry unit has a significant number of hospital-acquired patient pressure ulcers. Peggy, CNS, meets with a leadership team on the unit to discuss strategies to reduce pressure ulcers with the decision to explore using a unit-based turn team. Mary, staff RN, volunteers to work with Peggy on this project but expresses her concerns because she has never done a project such as this. Peggy develops a plan, then provides support and guidance by using evidence-based practice (EBP) with Mary. In addition, Peggy assesses, evaluates, and provides constructive feedback to Mary during the EBP process. At the conclusion of the EBP pilot, the findings show a significant reduction in pressure ulcers, so Peggy assists Mary to prepare and submit a poster for a national conference and it is accepted. This example illustrates how CNSs can support, guide best practices on the nursing unit, and encourage professional development for nursing staff. Being a CNS mentor to the nursing staff provides staff with the tools and skills to succeed in their work environment and nursing career.

WHAT IS THE DEFINITION OF MENTORING?

Katz (2001) describes mentoring as a personal and professional relationship characterized by mutual respect, trust, understanding, and empathy. An effective mentor is respected, reliable, patient, trustworthy, a very good listener, and a skilled communicator. CNSs have these attributes; therefore, CNSs are among the best mentors in a clinical setting. CNSs understand that their interactions with staff are opportunities to help them discover their potential at work and in their professional careers. A CNS has the opportunity, by mentoring staff, to directly affect the quality of patient care while simultaneously supporting patient safety and professional staff development.

This chapter discusses: (a) how you can develop a "mentoring perspective"; (b) what the essential qualities are for being a mentor; (c) what to consider when developing a mentoring plan; (d) misconceptions about mentoring; (e) "mentoring on the move" strategies; and (f) if you are already mentoring staff but had not realized it.

Developing a Mentoring Perspective

CNSs work in a variety of different settings, clinical areas, and specialties but all share a responsibility and commitment to serve as mentors to staff. Whereas health care has undergone many changes throughout the years, one CNS responsibility remains constant—the mentoring of staff. Mentoring is critical for staff nurses to succeed in the development of their professional careers; therefore, as a CNS, one of your most important responsibilities is to mentor staff. Not only do you serve as a role model to illustrate what it means to be a successful nurse, but also you serve as potential ally and advocate for all staff you encounter.

Does mentoring mean you will have to do mentoring duties in addition to the other responsibilities you already have? No, not at all. Mentoring is not a separate set of activities but rather it involves how you think and feel about yourself as a CNS and how you want to use your knowledge and expertise to help staff succeed. Most importantly, mentoring deals with how you, as a CNS, communicate with staff.

In addition, mentoring does not mean that you will have to spend huge amounts of time with individual staff members nor does it mean that you will have to mentor all new staff members whom you meet. What mentoring does mean is that you ensure each contact that you make with staff counts. It is not the quantity but the quality of time you spend with staff that sets mentoring apart from other kinds of activities. In other words, every time you meet a nurse there is a potential opportunity for mentoring. Separate meetings are not required to purposely act as a role model. Whatever setting or reason you have to talk with a nurse, through your words and actions you have the opportunity to serve as a mentor. Mentoring is a reciprocal relationship where both the CNS and staff benefit and learn from each other. As a CNS, you have the opportunity to make a difference in staff members' lives by serving as their mentor.

Essential Qualities for Being a Mentor

According to Butler and Felts (2006), the essential qualities of a mentor include: (a) nurturing the staff; (b) acting as a close, trusted, experienced clinical guide; (c) encouraging, teaching, and leading staff through significant points in their careers; (d) teaching by example; (e) acting as a sounding board; (f) giving honest feedback; and (g) helping the staff members to establish themselves in their profession. Trust and mutual respect are the basics of an active mentoring relationship because a trusting atmosphere is essential for meaningful communication to occur (Ibitayo, Baxley, & Bond, 2014). How do CNSs apply these mentoring qualities in the workplace?

The first quality, nurturing staff, is where CNSs provide support to staff in the clinical setting: (a) teaching about the "unwritten rules" of the unit, (b) introducing new staff to other staff, and (c) making new staff feel part of the team. Nurturing is providing a safe haven where staff members understand it is okay to ask questions. As a CNS, it is practicing unconditional acceptance of the nurse as a person while providing expert guidance on the necessary skills to work in a clinical area.

The second quality, acting as a close, trusted, and experienced guide, speaks to an essential component of the CNS's role—clinical expertise. Here is where your experience of doing a procedure "many times" really shines. The CNS can tell novice staff about those tips to make a procedure seem effortless. For example, a novice RN inserted a nasogastric (NG) tube but was not getting fluid return after it was connected to wall suction, so the RN called the CNS. Upon arriving at the patient's bedside, the CNS observed an anxious RN. The CNS then performed a quick assessment and discovered that the NG tube coiled in the patient's throat and removed it. Later, in a private setting, the CNS determined the RN's skill with NG tube insertion. The novice RN said, "I placed one NG tube as a nursing student but that was more than 2 years ago." The CNS concluded that the RN did not have sufficient knowledge and skills to insert the NG tube, so the CNS performed the procedure while creating a teachable moment. Two days later, the novice RN paged the CNS about another NG insertion. The CNS provided support and guidance with a plan where the CNS stood across the bed from the novice RN to explain to the patient, step by step, what will happen during the NG insertion procedure. The procedure steps were reviewed before entering the patient's room with the novice RN. While the RN set up the equipment, the CNS talked with the patient by saying, "Hi, my name is Peggy and I am a clinical nurse specialist who will be assisting Mary, your nurse, as she places the NG tube. What I want you to do is to listen to me as I tell you what is happening so you will know when to take a sip of water and hold your breath. Is this okay with you?" The patient says, "Yes." Peggy, CNS, had the patient's attention and cooperation as the nurse inserted the NG tube. The new nurse listened to what Peggy told the patient about what would happen next—real-time guidance. Once the NG insertion procedure was completed, the CNS and RN met briefly to evaluate the insertion procedure. In this scenario, the CNS demonstrated clinical expertise and guidance while mentoring staff competency and patient safety to create a win–win situation.

A third quality is guiding staff through important phases of their professional careers. Key points include: (a) provide an opportunity for staff to talk with you, (b) listen to a problem, (c) identify what needs to be done, and (d) provide resources. An example would be a graduate nurse who has taken the NCLEX licensing examination but did not receive a passing score. The CNS explores with the graduate nurse what factors may have contributed to the low NCLEX score and discovers that the graduate nurse becomes extremely anxious during examinations because they are timed tests. The CNS could suggest a NCLEX refresher class along with handouts or books on test-taking strategies to reduce testing stress and anxiety.

Teaching by example, the fourth quality, is an area in which a CNS excels. CNSs have been teaching since they first started their nursing careers. Almost daily, they teach patients about their medical conditions, families how to change a dressing, and other staff about new equipment. In addition, your CNS program provided you with knowledge about patient teaching that you used in your clinicals. When you think about it, you have been teaching your entire nursing career.

The fifth quality, acting as a sounding board, is an important quality for a CNS to use in the clinical setting. By understanding the clinical issues, you can help prepare the staff to succeed in its work environment. For example, join staff members in the break room and listen to what they are talking about and learn what their issues are.

Giving honest feedback creates a trusting relationship with staff. Nurses want to know about changes in their practice that affect quality care and patient safety. When staff discusses a clinical problem, consider sharing examples of an "I might do this" scenario to help staff learn about different ways to deal with the problem. As a CNS, you are the clinical innovation expert.

Finally, CNSs serve as role models for staff members when it comes to establishing themselves in their profession. Help them to find information about certification in a clinical specialty. If you are certified, share with them your experiences in preparing for your certification testing. Encourage members to belong to professional nursing organizations and help them find information.

Developing a Mentoring Plan

When mentoring staff, the CNS should develop a plan with measurable objectives. Here are four objectives to consider as you create your plan:

1. Establish a positive personal relationship with all staff members who you meet.
   - Make a proactive effort to act as a guide, a "coach," as well as an ally and advocate.
   - Trust and respect must be established. Be aware it takes time for staff to get to know you and how a CNS can help them. Take every opportunity to teach them about the CNS role and what you can do for them.
   - Regular interaction and consistent support are important in mentoring relationships. As you round, take time to stop and listen to members tell you about what is happening in their areas.
   - Once you have developed positive, personal relationships, it is much easier to realize the remaining three goals.
2. Help staff to develop career and life skills.
   - Work to accomplish specific goals for staff (e.g., staff's understanding of how to manage chest tube drainage systems).

When appropriate, emphasize critical-thinking skills such as decision making, goal setting, time management, dealing with conflict, and skills for coping with stress and fear (e.g., give them examples of how you managed your time as a staff nurse by sharing a story to which they can relate).

3. Assist staff in locating clinical and hospital resources.

Provide information or help your staff to find information about clinical resources (doctors, staff, policies and procedures, support services, professional organizations, etc.). Next, assist your staff in learning how to access and use these resources (e.g., sit down at a computer and show how to locate the on-line policy for blood transfusion, how to register for an on-line class).

4. Enhance your staff's ability to interact comfortably and productively with people from diverse racial, ethnic, cultural, and socioeconomic backgrounds.

As a CNS, your willingness to interact with people different from yourself will make a powerful statement about the values placed on diversity. Role-model the attitudes and behaviors that you emphasize (e.g., during rounds make time to talk with international nurses as well as new nurse graduates).

Acknowledge and understand cultural differences. Learn how to use differences as resources for growth to produce new understandings and insights. An international nurse told me, "It seems so lonely in American hospitals because some patients do not have family members with them at all times." Her comment reminded me to spend time and talk with those patients who have no visitors.

Work on understanding and critically examining your own perspectives on race, ethnicity, culture, class, religion, sexual orientation, and so on. Everyone holds preconceptions and stereotypes about one's own group and other groups. Take special care that you, as a CNS, are not (intentionally or unintentionally) promoting your views at the expense of your staff's viewpoints.

Consider virtual mentoring by using the Internet to interact with the mentee. Does the mentee have an e-mail address at work? Is there an intranet blog within the organization to make posts? And is Facebook a means by which one can communicate? This strategy could be used for setting up teaching scenarios or posting helpful tools for the staff.

Mentoring Misconceptions

When one thinks of a mentor, it conjures up certain unfounded beliefs about who is a mentor and what qualities mentors possess. Here are some mentoring myths:

Misconception: In a hospital, you need to be an older person with gray hair (or no hair) to be a good mentor.

Reality: In a hospital, mentors can be young or old. Some of the most outstanding mentors are your CNS colleagues regardless of age.

Misconception: Mentoring happens only one-to-one on a long-term basis.

Reality: In the health care setting, mentoring occurs in many different ways. Some mentoring relationships are traditional relationships involving a one-to-one relationship over a long period. However, effective mentoring can also occur in a group setting or even through a single encounter with a nurse. As a CNS, use each staff encounter as an opportunity for mentoring and think about ways to infuse mentoring into your daily work.

Misconception: Only a person being mentored benefits from mentoring.

Reality: By definition, mentoring is a reciprocal relationship where both the CNS mentor and the nurse learn from each other. True mentors are those who have developed the wisdom to learn from those they mentor.

Misconception: CNSs already have many responsibilities related to staff education and do not have the time to take on extra responsibilities related to mentoring.

Reality: Mentoring is not a separate set of activities that is different from any other job responsibility. Mentoring relates to the consciousness about one's work as a CNS and being a trusted ally for staff. Be a CNS who is staff centered and who can see and nurture the potential in others.

Misconception: By calling yourself a "mentor," you become a mentor.

Reality: Not all CNSs who work with staff are mentors, even if they have that job title. Mentors are those who have developed consciousness about mentoring and in their interactions with staff demonstrate respect, patience, trustworthiness, and strong communication skills, especially listening skills.

Misconception: To become a mentor requires a lot of time and work.

Reality: Becoming a mentor requires a change in consciousness; that is, how you think about yourself and how you think about others. Mentoring is not a matter of working harder or longer or adding to your job responsibilities but seeing your work differently.

Misconception: At a large hospital, one CNS can mentor only a limited number of staff. Although a CNS may want to help a large number of staff, the cold reality is that he or she can work only with a select few.

Reality: Each interaction with a staff member is a mentoring opportunity, every single encounter. The key is to develop consciousness about the importance of mentoring during your interactions with staff and to infuse this consciousness into your daily work as a CNS. In addition, it is important for CNSs to see themselves as part of a CNS network—as part of a community of mentors. To effectively help a particular nurse, a CNS mentor can draw upon this network or community. Mentoring occurs in a community, not in isolation.

Mentoring on the Move

"Mentoring on the move" describes ways the CNS can effectively mentor staff anywhere your work takes you. Here are some strategies to consider when you are mentoring on the move in your hospital:

- Include mentoring in daily staff interactions (e.g., rounding, at the nurse's station, helping with procedures).
- Mentoring occurs every day, in many forms and ways. Mentoring takes place in brief encounters that may have a powerful impact on a particular nurse.
- Mentoring works most effectively when it is done with purpose (e.g., teaching a new skill, collaborating on an evidence-based project, demonstrating use of new equipment, pursuing a common interest) but mentoring without a specific purpose can work too (e.g., being available as a sounding board).
- Issues related to diversity are key for CNSs. Sometimes diversity is viewed as a problem rather than an opportunity for enriching teaching and mentoring. For example, in a preceptor class, consider using a discussion panel of experienced RN preceptors, new graduate nurses, and international nurses. Have them share their perceptions of what it feels like to be in their roles.
- The timing of mentoring can be crucial. Mentoring may be needed after staff learn how to use new equipment or a new protocol (e.g., changing charting from paper to electronic requires frequent "on the spot" mentoring).
- Nurses who need the most mentoring are precisely those who "fall between the cracks" (e.g., staff who have not been trained on new equipment or a new protocol).

You Are Mentoring Staff When ...

Every day CNSs interact with staff, patients, families, physicians, and other health care workers throughout the hospital. Every time a CNS makes contact with another person, there is a potential mentoring moment. You are mentoring staff when you:

- Help staff members achieve potential within themselves that is hidden to others—and perhaps even to themselves.
- Share stories with staff about your own career and the ways you overcame obstacles that were similar.
- Help staff members overcome their fears of a coworker and help them to learn ways to deal with difficult personalities.
- Show staff how you learned time management when you worked as a staff nurse.
- Listen to a staff nurse describe a clinical problem and then explore resources at the hospital to help the staff nurse deal with the problem.

■ Help a new nurse understand a particularly tough procedure, and explain it in such a way that the nurse is willing to come back to you when there is another difficult skill to learn.

■ Know more about the staff nurse's clinical skills than what the nurse tells you.

SUMMARY

CNSs ensure patient safety, advance nursing practice, improve clinical outcomes, and provide clinical expertise to staff on a daily basis. CNS mentors are good listeners, approachable by nursing staff, committed to the nursing profession, and team players as well as role models for expert clinical practice (Modic & Schoessler, 2007). By incorporating the strategies described in this chapter into your practice, you realize the positive outcomes of your mentoring staff in your organization.

REFERENCES

Butler, M. R., & Felts, J. (2006). Tool kit for the staff mentor: Strategies for improving retention. *Journal of Continuing Education, 37*(5), 210–213.

Ibitayo, K., Baxley, S., & Bond, M. L. (2014). A positive culture brings success. *Nursing Management, 21*(3), 13.

Katz, S. (2001). Acceptance: A mentor's joy and responsibilities. *Pediatric Research, 49*(5), 725–727.

Modic, M. B., & Schlosser, M. (2007). Preceptorship. *Journal for Staff Development, 23*(4), 195–196.

CHAPTER 12

Precepting Students

GINGER S. PIERSON

The knowledge and skills needed to practice effectively as a clinical nurse specialist (CNS) continue to expand as medical, nursing science, and technological innovations seem to be almost continual. Additionally, nursing now offers multiple creative educational entry tracts into the nursing profession, which may create unique challenges and opportunities. CNSs must have the ability to both mentor and precept clinical staff and graduate students seeking advanced practice as CNSs. Nurses in both education and clinical practice must create workplace environments that support professional nursing practice. An important hallmark of professional practice is creating a nurse-to-nurse mentoring environment, where experienced nurses are encouraged to share their knowledge, skills, and enthusiasm about professional nursing practice with nurses who are less experienced (American Association of Colleges of Nursing, 2002). Mentoring and precepting activities serve to promote a continual climate of excellence and a culture of encouragement, acceptance, and support for building new skills (Firtko, Stewart, & Knox, 2005). Myrick and Yonge (2004) emphasize that "the relationship that evolved during the preceptorship experience was found to be pivotal not only to the enhancement of critical thinking, but also to the success of the experience and the student's own sense of professional competence" (p. 374). CNSs should embrace and practice critical thinking to foster growth in CNS graduate students as they learn the CNS advanced practice role and responsibilities.

Clinical currency and great flexibility/adaptability in CNS practice are highly valued and expected in your role and specialty. Clinical expertise within a specialty enables CNSs to provide expert advanced care to patients and clients to positively affect the delivery of care and resultant outcomes. These are often based on standards of care developed from best evidence-based practices (National Association of Clinical Nurse Specialists [NACNS], 2004). CNS skills are attained through extensive clinical experience as a bedside RN and then further developed as a CNS, with ongoing review of the literature for the latest evidence-based practices, networking with CNS colleagues, and active involvement in professional nursing organizations. These reflect some of the core components for effective CNS role development and implementation into practice. It is crucial to impart a foundation of these elements to CNS graduate students during their clinical preceptorship with advanced practice nurses, as CNSs implement their unique practice in very different ways and settings. Serving as a preceptor for graduate CNS students is a great honor and a professional responsibility. It carries with it accountability for thorough exposure to the role of the CNS. Time must be planned to show how the CNS role contributes to or impacts each of the three key spheres of influence: the patient/client sphere, the nurses/nursing sphere, and the system/organizational sphere (NACNS, 2004). Advance planning and ongoing discussion before and during the clinical rotation help define clear goals and direction for an effective CNS preceptor and CNS graduate student partnership. Five phases to serve as a guide for this partnership are discussed: becoming a CNS preceptor, defining the CNS/graduate student relationship and setting goals, active participation in the CNS role, professional association involvement, and evaluation of the clinical partnership experience.

BECOMING A CNS PRECEPTOR

You may want to consider spending your first year as a CNS in practice without precepting a graduate student. Time during this first year is needed for focused attention on adjusting to and refining the role/contributions within the organization as a CNS. This might be the first CNS role for the organization, or you may be replacing an experienced CNS with much history and expectation from the organization or units/patient populations served.

Once you are settled into the role of CNS, precepting a graduate may then seem possible and desirable. Discuss this commitment with your chief nursing officer or other appropriate supervisor to whom you report. Gain support for your planned preceptor and graduate student partnership, and consider how it will affect your role regarding time, projects, and plans for student involvement in all CNS activities and meetings. Involvement of other key nursing directors/leaders may also be necessary. This may include, for example, the director of nursing education, who may organize all nursing student academic contracts—including required school/hospital contract agreements, immunizations, background checks, confidentiality agreements, and more—prior to the student's start of the clinical rotation. Key aspects of hospital/nursing orientation, depending on the scope of the CNS practice/setting, may also be required for the graduate student prior to start of clinical. Most hospital organizations will welcome the opportunity of hosting graduate students, sharing in their clinical development and experience. This may also be an effective recruitment tool for future CNS positions for the organization.

Once organizational readiness has been obtained to host graduate students at your hospital/facility, contact the program chair of CNS graduate schools in your area and discuss serving as a clinical preceptor for graduate students. When the CNS clinical instructor contacts you, provide a detailed description of your experience as an RN, your experience as a CNS, and your current role responsibilities. This will provide the instructor with appropriate information to assign a graduate student to best develop an effective clinical partnership. Preceptor agreements and copies of your curriculum vitae or résumé are usually required for academic files.

DEFINING THE CNS/GRADUATE STUDENT RELATIONSHIP AND SETTING GOALS

The CNS preceptor and student relationship requires effective communication skills, trust, flexibility, and some interpersonal risk. Mutual respect fosters creative thinking and allows for achievement of high expectations of the CNS role. The role of the student is to accept responsibility for learning and to be actively engaged in the clinical experience with great interest and curiosity. The student should also have an ability to self-reflect on performance and accept and give feedback regarding the clinical experience (Butler & Felts, 2006).

Initial phone or e-mail contact is often established at least 1 to 2 months prior to the start of the clinical rotation. First priorities focus on completing required institutional contract requirements for the rotation and plans for any required hospital/nursing orientation. These should be discussed and dates for completion established. Further introductions are now necessary regarding each other's clinical experience as an RN and as a graduate student to find common ground for relating with each other. The student is always very interested in learning up front some details of your various functions and responsibilities as a CNS and how he or she may become involved. Care should be taken to not overwhelm the student with too much detail at the start, but just introduce broad responsibilities and projects of interest based on the student's background and anticipated class objectives.

Often during this initial phone or e-mail contact, the student has not started class yet and does not know details for the clinical rotation other than start and end dates, total number of clinical hours needed, and recommended number of clinical days per week to achieve the course goals. Specific objectives or projects that are required may not be known at this time. Initial dates for the first several clinical shifts are suggested at this time based on the CNS's schedule/availability. This may allow for further planning by the student, who may also have a work schedule to consider in addition to graduate school, family, and other commitments.

On the first day of clinical with the graduate student, an orientation plan should be created or reviewed for the clinical preceptorship, including plans for the evaluation process and the individual's learning style and preferences. A description of expectations for your CNS preceptor role and what is expected for the graduate student should be discussed and clarified. Dialogue during the clinical preceptorship should be ongoing between the CNS preceptor and the orientee. Feedback should be provided daily and progress discussed formally, often weekly or on a regular basis, throughout the preceptorship. Reassure the graduate student that any mistakes are kept confidential but reviewed to examine alternative decisions, actions, and possible outcomes (Modic & Harris, 2007). Immediate feedback is most productive and useful when reviewed just after the situation has occurred. This allows reflective thoughts at a time when recall is still fresh, honest, accurate, and relevant, and to correct and positively affect current knowledge and future clinical experiences (Brown, 2007).

Time should be allotted in the first 1 or 2 days together to review academic course objectives and required projects as they become known, as well as any further mutual expectations. One to 2 hours minimum is commonly needed to start this process. Further specific expectations to be discussed may include clinical hours to be spent and schedule flexibility as desired (more concentrated clinical for most weeks or spread out evenly over the entire rotation), a communication plan for absence or lateness for clinical, a plan for the best communication method between planned clinical shifts, professional behavior, confidentiality, communication and attire during clinical rotation, and expected follow-through on independent and collaborative projects.

During this first or second meeting, the student is often unsure of the expectations for the clinical course and tries to discover what the objectives/projects mean in terms of CNS clinical practice. Guidance is often needed to imagine and shape possible projects of interest to the student that also meet course objectives. Sharing ideas about key projects in which you as a CNS are involved helps at this early stage. Focus on those identified needs of your unit, patient population(s) served, or those needs related overall to the organization. This may help shape ideas for a brainstorming session for a follow-up meeting on the next clinical shift together. Identifying key project(s) early into the clinical rotation is critical to give the student time to get involved and complete, or greatly contribute to, a clinical project that is of mutual interest and will be clinically useful to both parties. If the right project is chosen, the student should feel excited to be involved with the project and, hopefully, feel proud when sharing this accomplishment or contribution with the faculty and other graduate students. These projects can be the start of developing a CNS portfolio of professional accomplishments and can be showcased in the interview process with future potential CNS employers. Additionally, the CNS graduate student should be encouraged to submit these completed projects to local and national CNS professional conferences as either posters or oral presentations to share ideas, strategies, and outcomes with other CNS colleagues. This creates early professional opportunities to present CNS accomplishments formally, facilitate networking with other CNSs, and spark interest and involvement in CNS organizations.

ACTIVE PARTICIPATION IN THE CNS ROLE
Exposure to All Aspects of the Role

When a CNS graduate student comes to gain realistic clinical experience as a CNS, the student should be allowed to become involved in and exposed to as many aspects of the CNS role as possible. No meetings, activities, projects, or other involvement should be avoided because of possible sensitivities that may exist in the organization. Examples of these potentially sensitive situations may include physician or RN peer review sessions, counseling of employees with directors (e.g., establishing clinical learning contracts), multidisciplinary sentinel and clinical event meetings, and The Joint Commission or Magnet® survey processes or regulatory agency reviews. The CNS may need to discuss and obtain permission (usually from the chief nursing officer) to have the student present at these meetings. Confidentiality agreements required for the organization may be signed by the student at the start of the clinical rotation. This agreement should cover any sensitive confidentiality concerns. Further discussions regarding expectations or limitations in sharing information with fellow students or faculty may also need to be addressed. Exposure to any or all of these situations allows the student to observe and discuss the role and contributions in each situation with the CNS. These are great learning experiences not to be missed. Be proactive as the CNS preceptor and look for these and other unique learning opportunities. The CNS and the graduate student should try to make an opportunity for a debriefing session following each meeting or regulatory survey. Discussion of overt/objective details covered in these meetings, as well as any subtle messages or interactions among team members, can provide valuable insight to the graduate student regarding group dynamics and navigating change in the organization.

Framework of Your CNS Role and Expectations

Providing a framework or overview of your CNS role, current projects, and activities early in the clinical experience can help the student gain perspective of the CNS role in practice. This may be reviewed in a written format (ideal) or discussed verbally. Include how each role component may be organized as affecting each of NACNS's three spheres of influence (NACNS, 2004). An overview will help give the student an idea of the multiple roles and responsibilities the CNS is frequently involved with and will help the student focus on the current responsibilities/role component(s) encountered within each clinical day. Obtaining a copy of the CNS job description and/or annual evaluation tool may help the student during this clinical rotation and future job interviews. Be sure to obtain permission from appropriate nurse leaders when sharing any organizational documents that may be considered sensitive or restricted by hospital/organizational policies. As clinical exposure of the CNS role grows, consider sharing how other CNSs in the organization, or other CNS professional colleagues, practice their roles differently; for example, unit-based CNSs, service-line-based CNSs, population-based CNSs, or other variations of CNS customer groups. Consider scheduling the graduate student with some clinical time (usually a half or full day) with these other CNS colleagues, as available, to see their various activities, settings, and the customers they impact.

Planning Clinical Days Together

Flexibility of clinical days, when possible, may be best matched to known, planned CNS activities of interest for the student, depending on availability for clinical. Graduate classes, work schedules, or family commitments may impact the schedule planned. Discuss availability or limitations to work night shifts, weekends, or other alternative hours. These may be regularly planned in the CNS schedule to provide CNS support to employees on all shifts as applicable to the CNS role. Scheduling several days together when time may be committed to focused clinical time on units/areas of responsibility is beneficial to prioritize. Additional time is also needed for discussion and work on clinical projects, for balancing ongoing time management of the CNS role, and for strategic planning. The CNS preceptor is expected to provide the daily clinical teaching with the graduate student but also has expectations from the unit/organization to meet CNS clinical practice expectations for the role (Burns, Beauchesne, Ryan-Krause, & Sawin, 2006). Ongoing planning and flexibility by all help achieve these responsibilities.

Active Clinical Involvement, Visibility, and Maintaining Clinical Currency

The CNS is known for clinical expertise and clinical currency, which helps give great credibility in serving as a resource and role model for nurses in a specialty. Establishing this expertise and credibility is critical to the success of the CNS role in the organization. Graduate students must see and understand this vital component of the many CNS functions. Clinical competency and currency are often most highly valued by the CNS's direct customers: nurses, patients/ families, and the organization. Working side by side with bedside nurses and sharing in all aspects of bedside care are especially important in the establishment of the perception/reality of CNS expertise, of the willingness to assist, and as a resource for all aspects of patient care related to the CNS's specialty area. This shared bedside care, involving the CNS and the staff nurse, allows the CNS to assess staff skills and develop a trusting and collaborative relationship. Maintaining clinical currency is reflected in assisted bedside practice in consultation roles, formal teaching of classes, informal teaching at the bedside, and in the identification and implementation of evidence-based clinical practice changes. Contributions involving the CNS's impact on clinical outcomes of patients and staff performance, on decreases in costs, and on patient length of stay are some of the many CNS role outcomes that may be measured to validate the direct CNS role contributions to the clinical areas of responsibility. The CNS must be actively involved in documenting leadership and participation in direct contributions to clinical excellence. Additionally, the CNS often provides leadership in applying evidence-based practice changes to clinical practice through formal organizational processes and use of change theory. Involvement of the student in the planning and implementation of an evidence-based practice project during the clinical experience can greatly help the transition of knowledge (evidence-based practice theory) into clinical practice.

Further discussion of the frequent struggle to balance maximal clinical time on the units supporting staff and patients, to manage time preparing and teaching formal classes, to work on multiple projects, and to take care of committee responsibilities is important to share with the CNS student. Sharing time-management strategies for the priorities most valued by the organization is crucial to the ongoing success of the CNS role and are discussed further in this chapter.

Work on Committees and Projects

Involvement of the student in ongoing committees may or may not be possible due to schedule conflicts, status of projects in process, or student preferences or interests. Much may be gained through attendance at committee meetings, such as the use of the CNS role in the committee; group dynamics, process, and politics; and evaluation of group leadership skills. These observations provide special opportunities for meaningful CNS dialogue for further role development of the student.

CNS's Education Role and Supportive Responsibilities

As previously mentioned, the CNS has an important role component in education—often in both formal teaching in the classroom and informal teaching done at the bedside with nurses and with patients and families. Some organizations/hospitals have nurse educators in separate supportive roles in addition to CNSs for specialty areas. An understanding of these separate, yet complementary, roles as well as their differences, or the addition of all educational responsibilities to the CNS role, is an important discussion to have with the graduate student. This helps the student understand role responsibilities for maintaining required education records, documentation of completed orientation and required initial clinical competencies, annual competency skills or knowledge validation for The Joint Commission or state regulatory agencies, and possible legal implications for the hospital in the future. When formal educator responsibilities are blended into the CNS role, reporting to a second director/manager for these educational responsibilities may also occur. Discussion of ongoing reporting responsibilities and expected communication, as well as issues of overtime compensation (if applicable) by department and assessment of annual/ongoing performance evaluation, may assist the student to explore and define expectations for future CNS interviews or job opportunities.

Prioritization of CNS Responsibilities and Time-Management Strategies

A student quickly learns during the clinical rotation that the CNS role is one of constant prioritization, time management, and required flexibility. As the CNS role is fully implemented and respected at the organization, multiple requests to involve the CNS's clinical expertise typically occur. Though viewed as a compliment to successful CNS role implementation and respect as a clinical expert, this can lead a CNS to be involved with too many educational classes or conferences, projects, committees, or other requests. This may also cause the CNS to lose focus on the highest priority CNS responsibilities, as too many tasks and requests are trying to be achieved simultaneously. One strategy that has proved effective for some CNSs has been to visibly post hospital/organizational/unit goals and strategic vision in the office. A regular evaluation of each CNS activity can be listed and compared with these strategic goals/vision to distinguish whether the activity supports this planned direction. Those activities that do not support the strategic goals/vision should be reevaluated and discussed as to the CNS's continued involvement in the commitment. A proactive list of each CNS activity, committee, and project as they are added to the CNS's workload can be a supportive strategy for a new or overwhelmed CNS. This list may include headings such as Routine Tasks, Responsive (Time-Limited) Tasks, or Strategic Planning and Support for Goals/Vision (Campbell, 2006). Ongoing additions to this list may help provide the CNS with an immediate evaluation of the task/project in relation to the outlined strategic direction and vision. This may help support the CNS's decision to decline involvement in requests or readily accept them for the right reasons. Refer to Chapter 7 for other strategies on this topic.

PROFESSIONAL ASSOCIATION INVOLVEMENT

CNSs need the opportunity to meet, support, and share ideas with other CNS colleagues regularly. Involvement with CNSs locally in the area may be possible within your hospital or clinic setting or in the surrounding community, whether formally as a CNS council or informally arranged by CNS colleagues with opportunities to meet as needed. Clinical specialty organizations may provide an opportunity to network with other CNS and RN colleagues both for clinical specialty and for CNS role development components.

Active involvement with the NACNS has provided a great deal of support for my role and growth as a CNS. Involvement in an NACNS committee and attending the annual NACNS conference each year are crucial priorities for networking with CNS colleagues at the conference and throughout the year via e-mail or phone, as desired. Graduate students should be encouraged to become involved with the professional nursing association for their clinical specialty and for CNS role development; they should become active members of NACNS to be well-rounded CNSs. Additional discussion of this topic is featured in Chapter 16.

EVALUATION OF THE CLINICAL PARTNERSHIP/EXPERIENCE

At the end of the clinical preceptorship with the graduate student, an evaluation is done of the achievement of planned goals, objectives, and student performance overall. This formal, written evaluation is supplied by the graduate student/program, often at the beginning of the clinical preceptorship. The tool should be reviewed together in the initial goal-planning stage and agreed upon as the evaluation that will be utilized to provide feedback. Sharing the completed evaluation or completing it with the graduate student may provide for effective feedback, including highlights of strengths identified in performance and opportunities for growth and further development. Honest feedback from the graduate student about the preceptorship experience at the facility, and with you as CNS preceptor/mentor for appropriateness as a preceptor, is also helpful for improvements for future CNS students (Stark, 2004). As RN and CNS colleagues, sharing this important information honestly and in a supportive manner is critically important for the growth of both persons. Mutual perceived achievement of assisting the graduate student in progressing toward becoming a safe, competent, compassionate, innovative, and collaborative CNS clinician would be a great outcome for your clinical preceptorship together (Burns et al., 2006).

SUMMARY

Serving as a CNS preceptor to graduate students has provided me with great professional and personal satisfaction over the years. By sharing with the new CNS colleague the successful CNS projects and strategies I have implemented, the times I have stumbled along the way, and the lessons learned from all of these experiences, I feel I am helping shape the future of CNS practice and the great contributions that can be made by each of us. I have always felt committed to precept, mentor, and guide other professional colleagues as a way to thank and honor all those nursing professionals who helped me be the CNS I am today. Following a plan, such as those outlined in this chapter, helps to keep your focus as a CNS on your established priorities and contributions to outcomes for patients, nurses, and the organization. This also allows for proactive or strategic planning and may facilitate preserving some of your time so that there is opportunity to precept graduate students and fully invite them into experiencing the CNS role. Much time and energy are often needed to precept students and we can feel overwhelmed with so many other demands for our time. Choosing your attitude as one of being positive and welcoming will greatly assist you and your student in having a great experience together for the clinical preceptorship. I have learned that CNS students are eager to learn, appreciate your valuable time and the energy you invest in them, and can contribute much if you let them. I still use today in my CNS practice many of the ideas, projects, and other contributions that graduate students developed during their clinical preceptorship. Many of these colleagues are successfully implementing their CNS roles in various settings and maintain a professional relationship with me. I enjoy every interaction I have with them and hope their experiences as students helped shape their current practice and that they too will help share the knowledge and skills gained with other professional colleagues in the near future.

REFERENCES

American Association of Colleges of Nursing. (2002, January). *AACN white paper: Hallmarks of the professional nursing practice environment.* Retrieved from http://www.aacn.nche. edu/publications/positions/hallmarks.htm

Brown, Y. (2007). Staff development story. *Journal for Nurses in Staff Development, 23*(5), 243–245.

Burns, C., Beauchesne, M., Ryan-Krause, P., & Sawin, K. (2006). Mastering the preceptor role: Challenges of clinical thinking. *Journal of Pediatric Health Care, 20*(3), 172–183.

Butler, M., & Felts, J. (2006). Tool kit for the staff mentor: Strategies for improving retention. *Journal of Continuing Education in Nursing, 37*(5), 210–213.

Campbell, G. (2006, March 16). *Defining success in the CNS role: An administrative perspective.* Presented at the NACNS Annual Conference, March 15–18, 2006. Salt Lake City, UT.

Firtko, A., Stewart, R., & Knox, N. (2005). Understanding mentoring and preceptorship: Clarifying the quagmire. *Contemporary Nurse, 19*(1–2), 32–40.

Modic, M., & Harris, R. (2007). Mastering precepting: Using the BECOME method to enhance clinical thinking. *Journal for Nurses in Staff Development, 23*(1), 1–9.

Myrick, F., & Yonge, O. (2004). Enhancing critical thinking in the preceptorship experience in nursing education. *Journal of Advanced Nursing, 45*(4), 371–380.

National Association of Clinical Nurse Specialists (NACNS). (2004). *Statement on clinical nurse specialist practice and education* (2nd ed.). Harrisburg, PA: Author.

Stark, S. (2004). Preceptor's expectations: An avenue to foster appropriate clinical experiences for advanced practice nursing students. *Journal of Continuing Education in Nursing, 35*(5), 234–235.

CHAPTER 13

Championing Evidence-Based Practice

DEBORAH J. SCHAFER

Evidence-based practice (EBP) has become one of the most significant and important principles in health care today. Some authors have declared that EBP is perhaps one of the most noteworthy themes to ever develop in global health care. The forces driving this paradigm shift are multifaceted and based on the recognition that many individuals do not receive research-based care, and that translating research into practice can lag by more than a decade (Hopp, 2014). The overarching role of all clinical nurse specialists (CNSs) is the delivery of safe, quality, cost-effective care. EBP methods impact every aspect of the CNS role— from direct care provider to consultant, from systems leader to collaborator, from researcher to advocate. The CNS is uniquely qualified and positioned to effect positive, sustained change for patients, nurses, and organizations alike through the work of knowledge transformation. As the intricacies of our health care environment become more complex, it is imperative that the CNS understands his or her role in the development and implementation of EBP, but of equal importance is the ability to articulate the knowledge, skills, and abilities necessary to bring this level of best practice to fruition. EBP is a composite of the triangle of best research, clinical expertise, and patient values. Full assimilation of these components into clinical decision making enhances the opportunity for delivery of the triangle of safe, quality, cost-effective care.

EBP OVERVIEW

Numerous definitions of EBP exist, but perhaps the most cited definition is the conscientious, explicit, and judicious use of current, best, research-based evidence when making decisions about patient care (Sackett, Strauss, Richardson, Rosenberg, & Haynes, 2000). The goal of EBP is to provide the most scientifically sound, high-quality care that reflects the choices and values of the patients we serve. It is a dynamic process that requires skill and vigilance to impact daily practice. A number of EBP models have been developed by nurse scientists to organize the steps of the EBP process, strengthen decision making, and help guide successful implementation of change. Commonly used frameworks include but are not limited to:

- Iowa Model of Evidence-Based Practice (Titler et al., 2001)
- Johns Hopkins Nursing Evidence-Based Practice Model (Dearholt & Dang, 2012)
- ACE Star Model of Knowledge Transformation (Stevens, 2004)
- ARCC (Advancing Research and Clinical Practice Through Close Collaboration Model; Melnyk & Fineout-Overholt, 2005)
- Stetler Model of Evidence-Based Practice (Stetler, 2010)

Each is based on a common five-step process: (a) formulation of a clinical question; (b) identification of pertinent research findings; (c) critical appraisal of relevant literature; (d) implementation of recommendations based on the evidence; and (e) evaluation of the outcomes. Using a framework leads to a systematic approach when undertaking EBP projects, and helps guide the advanced practice nurse in thorough development, implementation, and evaluation of the EBP process. Each model can be applied for extensive undertakings, but certain models may be better suited for your institution's needs and culture, so familiarize yourself with the different models and select the one best suited for your organization.

Although a well-executed EBP project is effective in identifying best practice, it does not guarantee meaningful transformation of that knowledge into practice. Bridging the gap of research and translation is complex, at times cumbersome, and requires proven strategies to implement and sustain practice and cultural change. Education alone is not sufficient to change behavior. Interventions need to be tailored based on the desired change and the impact that change will have on individuals and the organization. Successful assimilation occurs when evidence is strong, the environment is amenable to change, and the change process is appropriately facilitated (Hockenberry, Brown, & Rodgers, 2014). Effective change agents are detail oriented, focused on the big picture, and flexible to modifying ideas. They have the skills to articulate their vision and energize others. They have the ability to handle and manage resistance and are persistent in reaching their goals (Richardson, 2014). This step of practice integration may arguably be the one most dependent on the far-reaching skills of a CNS.

Evaluation is the final, but critical step in the EBP process. Both process and outcome measures are necessary in order to effectively analyze EBP initiatives. This can be difficult and/or expensive in the reality of a clinical setting. It is best to capture data that are clear, nurse-sensitive, and meaningful to the practice change and affected population. Analyzing the data for areas of accomplishment and opportunities for improvement will enable you to focus your efforts and resources in activities that will increase success and enhance outcomes. Sharing data on an ongoing basis, both positive and negative, is necessary in order to promote engagement and effect sustained change.

EXAMPLES OF SUCCESSFUL EBP PROJECTS

One of the goals of a CNS is to provide a therapeutic environment that addresses the complex needs of patients. Sometimes that requires the CNS to explore unconventional approaches to meet these challenges. That may be especially true in unique specialty populations. Long-term antepartum patients are hospitalized for weeks or even months due to complications of pregnancy. It is clear through both research and clinical experience that the effects of long-term bed rest and hospitalization on patients with high-risk pregnancies have significant negative physical and psychological ramifications. Studies report depression, anxiety, mood alterations, loneliness, and boredom. Many women express a sense of confinement and "being a prisoner" (Heaman and Gupton, 1998; Maloni, 1998; Richter, Parkes, & Chaw-Kent, 2007). While investigating strategies that could impact these patients, the CNS might discover that animals have been used for thousands of years in different cultures for therapeutic purposes. The benefits of animals in recovery from disease have been valued as far back as the time of Florence Nightingale. Animal therapy has demonstrated many physiologic and psychologic advantages. The presence of a dog aids in removing barriers to communication and in increasing social interactions by providing unconditional acceptance and breaking the tensions of hospitalization. Touching animals has been effective in relieving stress, improving coping abilities, and in reducing anger, hostility, tension, and anxiety. The mere presence of an animal in both short- and long-term environments is associated with decreased depression and effective reduction of loneliness, boredom, and isolation (Burch, 2003; Hooker, Freeman, & Stewart, 2002; Stanley-Hermanns & Miller, 2002). There is consistent evidence that human–animal interactions have a direct positive impact on health and happiness.

After a thorough literature search and critical appraisal of the research, the CNS might conclude that an animal therapy program could be a valuable avenue to address the emotional needs of long-term antepartum patients. One would first assemble a multidisciplinary group of all stakeholders including infection control, physicians (obstetric and maternal–fetal medicine), security, volunteer services, risk management, and legal affairs. Input should be elicited from the group in order to develop a clear, thorough policy and procedure for program implementation, as well as guidelines for the program coordinator and for handlers. The next step would be to focus on gaining support from administration, leadership, physicians, and nurses. The success of this step may hinge as much on the vigor of evidence as on the strength of the CNS's communication skills, especially when presenting such an innovative approach to care. The evidence and program proposal should be presented to all parties. Once support is gained, certified therapy dog teams are identified, and organizational volunteer requirements are met, visits may commence. Evaluations should be conducted for a period of time to ascertain patient response and overall value of the program. The CNS could create a simple Likert scale that measures therapy dog visit impact on satisfaction and emotion (happiness, anxiety, loneliness, depression, boredom). Evaluations might also collect information on whether a patient would recommend a visit for other patients, and if an animal therapy program would influence choice of a facility given the same level of care.

This particular example of an EBP project is simple in that it does not require substantial change to either physician or nursing practice. It might, however, depending on the philosophy of the organization, require a leap of faith and a cultural change in permitting such an innovative, nurse-driven approach to meet the needs of this unique population. The leadership, skilled communication, and commitment of the CNS would be essential to making this change a reality. The success would be attributed to (a) a thorough appraisal of the literature; (b) involving stakeholders early in the process; (c) developing a clear, thorough, and safe program based on research; (d) assessing and eliminating barriers; (e) disseminating evidence to engage staff; (f) monitoring implementation; (g) evaluating effectiveness; and (h) celebrating success.

Another more complex example of implementing evidence into practice might be that of developing a program to address obstetric hemorrhage. A major contributor to maternal morbidity, obstetric hemorrhage is a leading cause of maternal mortality. The incidence is rising and, tragically, most deaths are considered preventable. The risk of hemorrhage is always present in childbirth, and several strategies have been identified to improve the readiness, recognition, and response to hemorrhage that can minimize sequelae. The goal of a maternal hemorrhage EBP project should be to improve patient care by providing clear, thorough guidelines for practitioners to deliver swift, consistent, organized, seamless care that will decrease hemorrhage-related morbidity in women giving birth (California Maternal Quality Care Collaborative Hemorrhage Taskforce, 2009).

To begin, a thorough literature search should be performed. For "hot" issues such as this, an exhaustive literature search has often already been conducted by national think tanks. In addition, clear recommendations have typically been made to develop organization-specific evidence-based processes to address the issue. A multidisciplinary team including physicians (obstetrics, maternal–fetal medicine, anesthesia, intensive care unit [ICU] intensivist), nurses (antepartum, intrapartum, postpartum, ICU), administration, nursing leadership, quality improvement personnel, and laboratory/blood bank personnel should be assembled. Problem review including national- and organization-specific data should be presented, and a plan to move forward should be developed. A project of this magnitude demands the skill set unique to the advanced practice nursing role of a CNS to keep moving forward in a timely manner. A working group should meet frequently to review recommendations and available protocols, develop an institution-specific algorithm and order sets, formulate a multidisciplinary implementation plan that includes education and simulation, and define a post project outcomes measure strategy. Intermittent meetings should be held with all stakeholders to update project progress, gather information on potential barriers, and garner support for ongoing work. Unit and system approvals must be obtained for all order sets and protocols, as well as the implementation plan. The scope of such a project might require multi-layer implementation and easy-to-use guidelines for providers. Phase 1 might include (a) acceptance of an agreed-upon objective definition of hemorrhage; (b) implementation of an evidence-based risk assessment for hemorrhage; (c) application of a readiness protocol for patients at moderate or high risk of hemorrhage; and (d) data collection plan to measure risk assessment and protocol enactment. Phase 2 might encompass the development of an obstetric hemorrhage algorithm. This algorithm could include an initial-action nursing protocol, physician-driven order set, and massive transfusion order set. This phase should also include any tools or processes necessary to transform practice. For example, a medication kit that would allow one-step access to all medications potentially required to treat hemorrhage should be developed. Comprehensive instrument trays should be readily available for quick surgical intervention. Unit-specific equipment boxes that contain all supplies needed to promptly care for hemorrhage should be housed in a central location. Phase 3 might involve education and implementation of the algorithm. Education should be multidisciplinary, include additional instruction for unit champions to act as frontline experts, and consist of unit- and system-wide drills for obstetric massive transfusion simulations. Phase 4 should incorporate evaluation of project effectiveness and celebration of success. Meaningful evaluation metrics could include maternal hemorrhage risk assessment and lab readiness, ICU admissions related to hemorrhage, and blood administration of 5 or more units. Data should be shared with stakeholders and used to drive any necessary program revisions, as well as for ongoing monitoring of patient outcomes.

CLINICAL NURSE SPECIALIST ROLE IN EBP

It is evident that the full scope of the CNS role is required to successfully implement a comprehensive EBP program. Rarely does the work of a CNS impact just one patient, a single nurse, or a solitary process. Instead, the CNS improves care within a continuum by navigating through the three distinct spheres of influence of patient, nursing, and organizations. The core competencies of the role speak to the diversity and adaptability intrinsic to the role, which allows a CNS to have the widespread influence needed to make EBP changes. As a direct care provider, the CNS identifies gaps in knowledge and potential risks to patient safety and quality of care. She (I use this gender-specific pronoun only because most CNSs are female) acts as role model to ensure clinically competent care and develops cost-effective, efficient, evidence-based interventions to achieve patient or system outcomes. As consultant and collaborator, she works with others both within and across departments to design programs that meet clinical needs and promote clinical excellence. She mentors others in applying the principles of evidence-based care. She facilitates effective clinical teams through communication skills of coaching and guidance. The CNS remains current in research within her specialty. She identifies quality sources of data, understands statistical analyses, and draws conclusions of strength and applicability of literature. She fosters a spirit of clinical inquiry, designs effective programs of knowledge transformation, and integrates evidence into management of populations. As a system leader, the CNS navigates multiple disciplines and layers of bureaucracy to manage change. She uses effective strategies to empower others to influence clinical practice, change behavior, ensure a culture that demands best practice, and lead organizational change to improve outcomes through EBP. She disseminates outcomes achieved and communicates effectiveness of processes to organizational leadership, demonstrating the essential value of the CNS, thereby advocating for the role (National Association of Clinical Nurse Specialists [NACNS], 2010).

HOW TO GET STARTED

Your education has prepared you for the skills necessary to execute each step of an EBP project, but the only way to increase your knowledge and truly become expert is to immerse yourself in the process—each and every day. The task at hand can seem overwhelming, so here are a few helpful tips.

■ Refine your literature search skills. A well-developed search strategy saves time and elicits the most productive results. Depending on the literature database, your search terms may be searched exactly as entered or translated into a preferred terminology. Identify major themes and formulate keywords and related terms. Use a thesaurus if necessary. Use scientific terms and common names, and drug trade names and generics. For example, you may want to search sickle cell anemia, but related keywords include sickle cell disease, hemoglobin S disease or hemoglobinopathy. Another example is indomethacin. Try Indocin, nonsteroidal anti-inflammatory drug (NSAID), prostaglandin inhibitor, or tocolytic agent. Avoid multiword phrases, instead use "and" between words. Define a time period to search. Most recommend a 5-year span, but many valuable and even landmark studies can be missed by reducing the search to such a constricted time frame. Starting broad is often best. You can narrow the exploration by adding or refining terms until you have tapered the search sufficiently to produce the best literature for the question at hand. Each database has unique characteristics, so it simply takes practice to determine the best search terms and approach. Also remember the importance of indexing. If you use the search term "labor," did you want articles on labor, meaning "to work" or did you want information on giving birth? Or is it "labour?" Indexing expedites more precise search strategies, especially for terms that are broad or vague. Truncation strategies allow you to search for variant word endings. Geno* will pick up genome, genomics, and genotype. Be careful not to truncate a word too early, as this will retrieve many related as well as unrelated words. Finally, remember that librarians are your friends! They are invaluable in assisting you to shape your search tactic or finding appropriate studies that somehow just elude you.

- Hone your critical appraisal skills. Review and critique quantitative and qualitative research studies, as well as systematic reviews and clinical guidelines. Always use tools appropriate for the literature you are reviewing. Tools help to identify methodological strengths and weaknesses and provide consumers of research evidence the opportunity to make informed decisions about the quality of the science.
- Facilitate journal clubs. These forums serve to educate and enlighten all participants to the chosen topic, and are a great way to further enhance your literature evaluation skills. They also help ignite passion in both you and your bedside nurses about a specific practice issue.
- Conduct clinical inquiry rounds. Ask nurses to identify relevant clinical issues. Cultivate an environment that encourages and rewards the pursuit of knowledge and one that consistently asks the questions: Why do we do this? or Is this the best way to reach this outcome? Help the staff frame the question in a searchable manner—population, intervention, comparison intervention, and outcome (PICO). Encourage and assist the nurse to find evidence that answers the question.
- Chair a practice council and establish an expectation that practice is based on evidence rather than tradition. Routinely review policies, procedures, management guidelines, and protocols. Ascertain that these resources are based on sound science, or revise them to reflect best practice.
- Offer presentations about EBP. This can be accomplished through formal lectures or informal monthly workshops. A variety of venues is suitable for such information including nursing grand rounds, RN residency programs, EBP fellowships, college-level nursing classes, or programs for local chapters of specialty nursing organizations.
- Partner with an academic institution to promote EBP and research skills in both nurses and nursing students. One innovative program, Research Roundtable (Harne-Britner & Schafer, 2009), described the collaborative partnership between a community health care system and a local baccalaureate nursing program. The program paired bedside nurses with senior-level nursing students to examine clinical problems through the EBP process. The group met seven times throughout the semester to systemically develop a researchable question, search and evaluate the literature, and make recommendations based on literature. Nursing faculty and seasoned CNSs mentored clinical educators and novice CNSs. Group facilitators guided and coached bedside nurses and students. A distinct advantage of this partnership was the synergy among nurses'

clinical practice expertise, the students' information management and general computer skills, and the faculty and facilitators' knowledge of research and EBP. All participants gained valuable, meaningful knowledge of the EBP process, and patients ultimately reaped the benefits of best practice. The health care organization realized successful EBP changes or completed research studies generated through this initiative. The college ultimately revised its curriculum to include a course dedicated entirely to EBP.

- Familiarize yourself with the EBP process. There are many excellent websites, books, and articles that are informative and helpful in guiding you along each step of the journey. The American Nurses Association's (ANA) Research Toolkit is a great place to start. It offers resources to guide you through the process, from searching the literature to translating the evidence to shaping health policy (ANA, 2012). A series of 11 articles written by the Arizona State University College of Nursing and Health Innovation's Center for the Advancement of Evidence-Based Practice provides step-by-step guidance in implementing EBP. The series begins with igniting a spirit of inquiry (Melnyk, Fineout-Overholt, Stillwell, & Williamson, 2009) and ends with evaluating and disseminating the impact of an evidence-based intervention (Fineout-Overholt, Gallagher-Ford, Melnyk, & Stillwell, 2011).
- Start with a simple EBP project. Choose an issue about which you are passionate—one that has the potential to make real and positive change in the outcomes of your patients. The focus should be small in scale and one that will impact a single unit or a small population group. This will build your skills and confidence with each step, and will help to keep the project execution and timetable manageable.
- Choose the EBP model best suited for your organization. Conduct your project using the chosen model. Do not skip steps or dismiss steps as unimportant. The model offers a systematic guide in helping to ensure the thoroughness of approach and ultimately the success of the project. Consider using a checklist to keep you on track (Table 13.1).
- If possible, work with a mentor. That person can act as a sounding board through each of the steps, offer assurance that you are on the right track and guidance when needed, help you navigate some of the trickier avenues in project implementation, or simply serve as a cheerleader along the way.
- Once you have successfully completed this first project, you will feel better prepared to tackle larger, broad-based, system-wide projects.
- After all that, it will be your turn to act as a mentor to ambitious bedside nurses or novice CNSs as they undertake their first EBP project. There is little that rivals the sense of fulfillment you feel when mentoring the professional growth of others through skilled guidance and encouragement.

TABLE 13.1 Checklist for Evidence-Based Practice (EBP)

1. Phrase the research question in a way that will increase the likelihood of finding the most appropriate literature to answer the question.
2. Perform a thorough literature search.
3. Utilize appropriate tools to critically appraise the type of literature found.
4. Summarize findings focused on practice implications.
   a. Determine if evidence is sufficiently sound or compelling to merit a practice change.
   b. Perform additional literature search if needed.
5. Formulate a detailed plan for implementation of evidence.
   a. Identify and include all stakeholders.
   b. Discuss known/potential barriers of implementation and strategies to minimize obstacles.
   c. Secure approval, support, and necessary resources for practice change (system/unit leadership).
   d. Develop educational and roll-out plan.
6. Create plan for evaluation of outcomes.
   a. Collect pre implementation/baseline data whenever possible.
   b. Include data measures, methods, sources, collectors, frequencies, and dissemination.
   c. Select outcome measures that clearly reflect successful project implementation.
7. Launch EBP
   a. Consider piloting change on key units if the proposed practice change is broad in scope.
   b. Be readily available during initial implementation phase.
8. Review/revise implementation plan as needed.
   a. Meet with stakeholders to examine progress and report outcomes.
   b. Discuss successes, opportunities for improvement, issues, and unforeseen barriers.
   c. Strategize avenues to maintain/enhance success.
9. Disseminate your results.
   a. Discuss project in depth, including lessons learned.
   b. Present project at local/state/national venues or via professional publication.

SUMMARY

This chapter was created to reinforce the integral role of the CNS in the EBP process, and to offer practical strategies to enhance success along the way. EBP has become the buzzword phrase of health care systems to provide quality care.

Patients demand care based on science and health care organizations are obligated to provide the best care. But redesigning care delivery processes does not occur without expert, multifaceted skills—the very attributes of a CNS. The call for EBP allows the CNS to improve delivery of safe care, positively impact quality outcomes, and establish a vital presence within the organization.

REFERENCES

American Nurses Association. (2012). *Research toolkit*. Retrieved from http://nursingworld .org/Research-Toolkit

Burch, M. R. (2003). *Wanted! Animal volunteers* (revised ed.). New York, NY: Howell Book House.

California Maternal Quality Care Collaborative Hemorrhage Taskforce. (2009). *California Maternal Quality Care Collaborative toolkit to transform maternity care*. Retrieved from www.cmqcc.org

Dearholt, S. L., & Dang, D. (2012). *Johns Hopkins nursing evidence-based practice model and guidelines* (2nd ed.). Indianapolis, IN: Sigma Theta Tau International.

Fineout-Overholt, E., Gallagher-Ford, L., Melnyk, B. M., & Stillwell, S. B. (2011). Evaluating and disseminating the impact of an evidence-based intervention: Show and tell. *American Journal of Nursing, 111*(7), 56–59.

Harne-Britner, S., & Schafer, D. J. (2009). Clinical nurse specialists driving research and practice through research roundtables. *Clinical Nurse Specialist, 23*(6), 305–308.

Heaman, M., & Gupton, A. (1998). Perceptions of bed rest by women with high-risk pregnancies: A comparison between home and hospital. *Birth, 25*(4), 252–258.

Hockenberry, M. J., Brown, T. L., & Rodgers, C. C. (2014). Implementing evidence in clinical settings. In B. M. Melnyk & E. Fineout-Overholt (Eds.), *Evidence-eased practice in nursing healthcare: A guide to best practice* (3rd ed., pp. 202–223). Philadelphia, PA: Wolters Kluwer Health.

Hooker, S., Freeman, L., & Stewart, P. (2002). Pet therapy research: A historical review. *Holistic Nursing Practice, 17*(1), 17–23.

Hopp, L. (2014). Shaping practice: Evidence-based practice models. In J. S. Fulton, B. L. Lyon, & K. A. Goudreau (Eds.), *Foundations of clinical nurse specialist practice* (2nd ed., pp. 145–162). New York, NY: Springer Publishing Co.

Maloni, J. A. (1998). Antepartum bed rest: Case studies, research and nursing care. *AWHONN Symposium*. Association of Women's Health, Obstetric and Neonatal Nurses, Washington, DC.

Melnyk, B. M., & Fineout-Overholt, E. (2005). *ARCC: Advancing research and clinical practice through close collaboration*. Gilbert, AZ: ARCC Publishing.

Melnyk, B. M., Fineout-Overholt, E., Stillwell, S. B., & Williamson, K. M. (2009). Igniting a spirit of inquiry: An essential foundation for evidence-based practice. *American Journal of Nursing, 109*(11), 49–52.

National Association of Clinical Nurse Specialists. (2010). *Clinical nurse specialist core competencies*. Retrieved from http://www.nacns.org/docs/CNSCoreCompetenciesBroch.pdf

Richardson, J. (2014). Managing the change/innovation process. In J. S. Fulton, B. L. Lyon, & K. A. Goudreau (Eds.), *Foundations of clinical nurse specialist practice* (2nd ed., pp. 81–96). New York, NY: Springer Publishing Co.

Richter, M. A., Parkes, C., & Chaw-Kent, J. (2007). Listening to the voices of hospitalized high-risk antepartum patients. *Journal of Obstetric, Gynecologic and Neonatal Nursing, 36*(4), 313–318.

Sackett, D. L., Strauss, S. E., Richardson, W. S., Rosenberg, W., & Haynes, R. B. (2000). *Evidence-based medicine: How to practice and teach* EBM (2nd ed.). London, UK: Churchill-Livingstone.

Stanley-Hermanns, M., & Miller, J. (2002). Animal-assisted therapy: Domestic animals aren't merely pets. To some, they can be healers. *American Journal of Nursing, 102*(1), 69–76.

Stetler, C. B. (2010). Stetler model. In J. Rycroft-Malone & T. Bucknall (Eds.), *Models and frameworks to implementing evidence-based practice: Linking evidence into action* (pp. 51–82). Oxford, UK: Blackwell Publishing Limited.

Stevens, K. R. (2004). *ACE Star Model of EBP: Knowledge transformation.* Academic Center for Evidence-based Practice. San Antonio, TX: The University of Texas Health Science Center at San Antonio. Retrieved from www.acestar.uthscsa.edu

Titler, M. G., Kleiber, C., Steelman, V., Rakel, B. A., Budreau, G., Everett, L. Q., … Goode, C. J. (2001). The Iowa model of evidence-based practice to promote quality care. *Critical Care Nursing Clinics of North America, 13*(4), 497–509.

PART IV

EVALUATION

CHAPTER 14

Documenting Clinical Outcomes

DEBORAH G. KLEIN

Increased demand for accountability, ongoing changes in health care delivery, focus on improving outcomes, and changing reimbursement have pushed clinical nurse specialists (CNSs) to verify their contributions and demonstrate their value. Greater focus on outcome measurement is evident with mandatory reporting of hospital quality measures. CNSs are expected to lead in collecting and using clinical, economic, and quality outcomes data. Evidence of CNS impact occurs in many ways, including outcome measurement activities, process improvement analyses, cost avoidance and cost savings activities, and program evaluation. The *Statement on Clinical Nurse Specialist Practice and Education* (National Association of Clinical Nurse Specialists [NACNS], 2004) outlines core competencies and essential characteristics of CNS practice that produce outcomes. These core competencies were revised and published by NACNS in 2010 (National CNS Competency Task Force, 2010). Achievement of these outcomes is driven by individual interest, availability of financial and material resources, expectations of the institution, organizational culture, and support of others. Even the new CNS must consider ways to demonstrate his or her impact on clinical outcomes.

The new CNS must often demonstrate that clinical expertise before he or she can impact clinical outcomes (Klein, 2007). However, with strong clinical leadership skills, including open-mindedness, professional demeanor, mentoring, and excellent communication skills, a new CNS can impact clinical outcomes while demonstrating clinical expertise. The ability of the CNS to recognize patterns in resource utilization and care delivery processes makes the CNS an ideal facilitator of quality improvement activities in which data can direct and support decisions on how to achieve best practices (Duffy, 2002; Finkelman, 2013; Ingersoll & Mahn-DiNicola, 2005; Sparacino & Cartwright, 2009). System inefficiencies, obstacles to continuity of care, and the inability of others to see the "big picture" can be identified through pattern recognition.

Three phases have been described that serve as a framework for the development of an effective outcome evaluation plan that any CNS can use (Ingersoll & Mahn-DiNicola, 2005). The first phase is defining the core questions that need to be answered; the second phase is defining the data required to answer the questions; and the third phase focuses on deriving meaning from the data and acting on the result (Box 14.1).

PHASE I: DEFINE THE CORE QUESTION

Defining the core question is the foundation for developing an effective outcome plan. As part of this process, the CNS must ensure that the question clarifies the purpose and the goals of the CNS within the organization. The CNS should discuss with the nurse manager or administrator the role expectations to ensure that they are reasonable and appropriate. Attempts should be made to focus on nurse-sensitive outcomes (patient falls, ventilator-associated pneumonia, skin breakdown) rather than areas where the CNS may have an impact (decreasing length of stay, decreasing hospital costs; Doran, Sidani, & DiPetro, 2014). The new CNS must ensure that the question is simple and able to be successfully answered. By successfully addressing a clinical practice concern, the new CNS will gain credibility and respect.

Questions can come from CNS observations of clinical practice, quality data, or directly from the nursing staff. The nurse manager may approach the new CNS with a clinical issue that needs further development; for example, strategies to reduce patient falls, effectiveness of pain management, evaluating

---

Box 14.1 Outcome Evaluation Planning Process

Phase I: Define the core question
1. Clarify the question
2. Define the population to be evaluated
3. Identify the stakeholders
4. Review the literature
5. Identify interventions
6. Develop the core question

Phase II: Define the data elements
1. Identify the population
2. Establish performance and outcome measures or indicators
3. Identify and evaluate the data

Phase III: Derive meaning from data and act on results
1. Analyze data and interpret results
2. Present and disseminate findings
3. Identify improvement opportunities
4. Develop a plan for implementation and reevaluate

Adapted from Ingersoll and Mahn-DiNicola (2005).

documentation of restraints, or examining skin breakdown rates. Although the new CNS may not desire to focus on these issues, selecting one of these areas for process improvement is an effective way to demonstrate cooperation, collaboration, and credibility, and to earn trust and respect.

One of the most important areas in which the CNS has value is in helping to ensure that evidence-based practice changes are implemented. Several national quality and safety measures have been published that focus on high-volume, high-risk populations and can serve as guides for developing CNS outcome evaluation plans. Some of these measures include the National Patient Safety Goals for Hospitals from The Joint Commission, National Quality Improvement Goals—Oryx Performance Core Measures from The Joint Commission, National Quality Forum, Agency for Healthcare Research and Quality of the Department of Health and Human Services, Institute of Medicine's 5 Million Lives Campaign, Surviving Sepsis Campaign, and The Leapfrog Safe Practices Score. The new CNS can refer to any one of these sources for identifying potential questions.

The next step is to define the population to be evaluated. Many CNSs perform a variety of activities with heterogeneous populations in their clinical practice. Therefore, it is necessary for the CNS to focus on specific aspects of practice with a specific patient group. This focus helps create a more manageable and successful outcome plan and limits extraneous variables that could interfere with the interpretation of the findings. For example, the new CNS should consider limiting the population to one unit (e.g., the surgical intensive care unit [ICU]) or a specific aspect of a diagnosis (e.g., diabetic patients with foot ulcers seen in an outpatient clinic). If possible, the target population should be comparable to other groups monitored through quality improvement activities at the organizational or departmental level.

The CNS must also identify the stakeholders in the process. The CNS is often the individual facilitating the team, and early identification of the stakeholders will facilitate the design of the outcome evaluation. Stakeholders may include nursing staff, the nurse manager, physicians, pharmacists, and other members of the health care team. Encouraging their participation early on, incorporating their ideas, and providing updates throughout the process will help clarify the CNS role to them and have them acknowledge the new CNS as a valuable member of the team. Together these individuals become the process team.

The nurse manager of the patient care area is responsible for ensuring that the unit has the needed resources, that staff has the necessary skills and knowledge to perform its jobs, and that the environment supports the staff in delivering care and meeting organizational goals (Disch, Walton, & Barnsteiner, 2001). The CNS can support these nurse manager responsibilities, and together the CNS and the nurse manager can develop a strong partnership in ensuring that nursing standards form the basis of nursing practice. It is imperative that the nurse manager support the outcome evaluation plan. Not only will the CNS benefit, but the desired outcomes will impact nursing practice on that unit. In many instances, it may be the nurse manager who identifies an outcome project for the new CNS.

The final step is to review the literature for current standards of care, regulatory requirements, national guidelines, and established or emerging evidence-based best practices that are relevant to the question. Outcome data already available in an institution should also be considered, as these will save time, energy, and money (Gawlinski, 2007). Using this information, interventions can be identified, which may include a new documentation tool, patient education materials, or the development of a new process to ensure patient safety. Once goals and interventions are identified, the core question can be developed. Ingersoll and Mahn-DiNicola (2005) have formulated some basic questions that can be useful to help establish the outcome evaluation plan (Box 14.2). Once the core questions are determined by the CNS and other members of the process team, the data collection method can be designed.

PHASE II: DEFINE THE DATA ELEMENTS

There are three steps in defining the data elements: identify the population, establish performance and outcome measures or indicators, and identify and evaluate the data. This phase is often challenging for the new CNS, particularly if the CNS has had little exposure to quality improvement principles and management information systems, both of which support outcome evaluation. The CNS should seek assistance from other health care professionals who have experience in continuous quality improvement principles, health care statistics, nursing informatics, or program evaluation.

Box 14.2 Questions That Can Be Used in Creating an Outcome Evaluation Plan

How cost-effective is this program?

How satisfied are patients with the service they receive?

How closely does the health care team adhere to best-practice standards?

What are the barriers that influence the ability of the staff to carry out the practice?

How many patients have complications of care?

What patient safety issues associated with this population should be examined?

What can be done to reduce resource utilization for this population?

What needs to be done differently in order to become a center of excellence for this population?

How can the CNS contribute to the training and development of other staff?

Adapted from Ingersoll and Mahn-DiNicola (2005) and Gawlinski (2007).

Although identifying the population may seem obvious, it is important to determine inclusion criteria. This will serve as the denominator for the specific indicator, which is typically a number, rate, or sum. For example, it may be easier to study interventions that decrease the incidence of ventilator-associated pneumonia in intubated patients on mechanical ventilation in *one* ICU as the target population than to include all intubated patients on mechanical ventilation in *several* ICUs.

Establishing performance and outcome measures or indicators involves determining which data will be collected to answer the core question. The CNS should consider data available from national database services for benchmarking. Indicators can include readmission rates for a specific diagnosis, patient fall rate per 1,000 patient days, central line associated bloodsteam infections per 1,000 line days, or average length of stay. A draft list of indicators should be created and shared with the team for feedback and suggestions. Achieving team support of the indicators is imperative for the CNS to be perceived as being able to successfully answer the core question and therefore be effective in the CNS role.

The new CNS must be aware that he or she may be asked to collect data for other health care providers that have little to do with the CNS's ability to influence care. For example, interventional cardiologists are interested in the time from the first incision for patients undergoing stent placement to the time the wire crosses the lesion in the coronary artery. The CNS has no role in influencing this process, and it should not be part of a CNS outcome plan. The CNS can, however, identify other potential resources that may be available to gather this information. The CNS must stay focused on goals for which he or she is responsible.

The final step is identifying and evaluating the data elements. A new CNS may consider using short-term outcome measures, such as blood glucose levels, pressure ulcer development, or patient falls, instead of long-term outcomes measures, such as readmission rates, return clinic visits, or length of stay (Byers & Brunell, 1998). The details of the data collection tools and the actual data collection process are examined: How easy is the instrument to use? How much time does it take to complete? Is this tool useful in determining the effect of the CNS in nursing practice? Whenever possible, it is easier to use instruments already established rather than to develop new ones. The data collection instrument should be short, concise, user friendly, and easy to complete.

To help the CNS determine which indicators are essential versus those that are interesting but not essential, the CNS can list each indicator on a piece of paper and then write down all aspects of data collection for each indicator. For example, if determining a rate, definitions of the numerator and denominator and the source for each data element are listed. Hospital management information systems can be a source of data. Risk management systems can provide details of medication errors, transfusion reactions, or other adverse outcomes. Pharmacy systems may track the time when first dose of a specific medication was administered or the number of doses of a specific medication a patient received. Laboratory, radiology, and clinical documentation systems can also provide needed data. Experts are available to assist in retrieving data from these systems.

Outcome indicators should be measured before (at baseline) and after the practice change. Measurement at these times allows a before-and-after comparison of the effects of the practice change.

Once the indicators and data elements have been finalized and the data sources determined, the CNS should summarize the outcome evaluation plan in a concise document. Timelines and who is responsible for data collection and data analysis are included. Documenting the plan in this manner simplifies implementation and clarifies the responsibility of all participants. This document is shared with the process team to ensure support.

PHASE III: DERIVE MEANING FROM DATA AND ACT ON RESULTS

The final phase of the outcome evaluation plan process includes analyzing, evaluating, and disseminating the findings, along with identifying opportunities for improvement. The goal is to improve quality, cost, and customer satisfaction, and to evaluate the contributions of the CNS.

The CNS may be responsible for data analysis; however, including others (e.g., a statistician or doctorally prepared nurse researcher) in the process may help eliminate any perceived bias. The resulting data can be compared with baseline information or a known standard of care or benchmark.

Findings, conclusions, and recommendations for future practice are essential components of the outcome evaluation process. The way the findings are presented will depend on the personnel receiving the information. Generally, charts or tables are an effective way to present data. Control charts display performance data against upper and lower control limits that reflect normal variation in a system. Data lying outside the upper and lower limits and clusters of data within the limits indicate variations that require further investigation (Burns & Quatrara, 2013).

Control charts can also document processes over time. For example, it was noted that, despite the implementation of an insulin infusion protocol and preprinted order set in an ICU, blood glucose levels were not within the expected range 60% of the time. The CNS led a team of staff nurses, a nurse manager, a pharmacist, and the medical director of the ICU in developing and implementing a process to move blood glucose levels into the expected range. Data for the control chart were used to show meaningful changes that occurred as a result of the CNS's efforts (Figure 14.1). The longitudinal display of data provides an accurate and informative representation of the CNS's impact than would be seen by a simple comparison of average blood glucose levels before and after the intervention.

Once the findings have been prepared for review, they must be interpreted and potential opportunities for improvement identified. This process is similar to any work design initiative. Champions and potential opponents of change

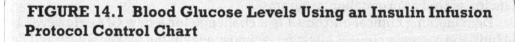

FIGURE 14.1 Blood Glucose Levels Using an Insulin Infusion Protocol Control Chart

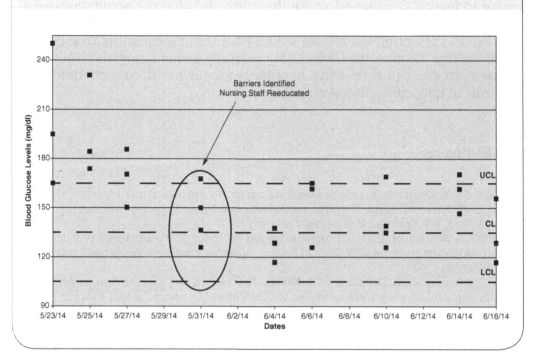

should be identified. Specific goals and interventions are developed as well as the level of difficulty with implementing the change, projected costs, and the human and technological resources required to implement and sustain the change. The CNS must consider how much time will be involved in this project and how it may affect other areas of practice. For example, if the goal of the performance improvement plan is to maintain the patient's blood glucose levels between 140 and 180 mg/dL, interventions might include reeducating the nursing staff in the ICU on the insulin infusion protocol to ensure that it is initiated at the appropriate time. Although the time commitment to review the insulin infusion protocol with 60 RNs will be great, the benefit to the patient will be even greater. In addition, it will help establish credibility for the new CNS.

Once goals and strategies to meet these goals have been established, they should be summarized and distributed to the process team as well as to the nursing staff and attendees of department meetings. Each goal should specify the primary intervention that will be used to reach the goal as well as who is accountable for the actions required and the target dates for completion. The CNS can then use this established plan to reevaluate the outcome, which can then be used as the basis for future outcome evaluation plans. Other strategies to ensure that practice changes are sustained include incorporating them into institutional documents such as policies, procedures, guidelines, and competencies as well as orientation programs.

Documenting clinical outcomes is a challenge for a new CNS. However, by identifying a simple clinical question, acknowledging the stakeholders and listening to their ideas, reviewing the literature, defining the population, establishing the outcome indicators, collecting and analyzing the data, interpreting the results, presenting the results with a plan for implementing changes, and implementing the plan, the CNS can successfully demonstrate his or her value. These strategies can then serve as a basis for further documentation of the CNS role in impacting clinical outcomes.

REFERENCES

Burns, S. M., & Quatrara, B. (2013). Selecting advanced practice nurse outcome measures. In R. M. Kleinpell (Ed.), *Outcome assessment in advanced practice nursing* (pp. 73–91). New York, NY: Springer Publishing Company.

Byers, J. F., & Brunell, M. L. (1998). Demonstrating the value of the advanced practice nurse: An evaluation model. *AACN Clinical Issues: Advanced Practice in Acute and Critical Care, 9,* 296–305.

Disch, J., Walton, M., & Barnsteiner, J. (2001). The role of the clinical nurse specialist in creating a healthy work environment. *AACN Clinical Issues: Advanced Practice in Acute and Critical Care, 12,* 345–355.

Doran, D. M., Sidanai, S., & DiPietro, T. (2014). Nurse sensitive outcomes. In J. S. Fulton, B. L. Lyon, & K. A. Goudreau (Eds.), *Foundation of clinical nurse specialist practice* (pp. 41–64). New York, NY: Springer Publishing Company.

Duffy, J. R. (2002). The clinical leadership role of the CNS in the identification of nurse-sensitive and multidisciplinary quality indicator sets. *Clinical Nurse Specialist, 16,* 70–76.

Finkelman, A. (2013). The clinical nurse specialist: Leadership in quality improvement. *Clincial Nurse Specialist, 27,* 31–35.

Gawlinski, A. (2007). Evidence-based practice changes: Measuring the outcome. *AACN Advanced Critical Care, 18,* 320–322.

Ingersoll, G. L., & Mahn-DiNicola, V. A. (2005). Outcome evaluation and performance improvement. In A. B. Hamric, J. A. Spross, & C. M. Hanson (Eds.), *Advanced practice nursing: An integrative approach* (pp. 875–941). St Louis, MO: Saunders Elsevier.

Klein, D. G. (2007). From novice to expert: CNS competencies. In M. McKinley (Ed.), *Acute and critical care clinical nurse specialists: Synergy for best practices* (pp. 11–28). St Louis, MO: Saunders Elsevier.

National Association of Clinical Nurse Specialists (NACNS). (2004). *Statement on clinical nurse specialist practice and education* (2nd ed.). Harrisburg, PA: Author.

National CNS Competency Task Force. (2010). *NACNS core competencies.* Retrieved from http://www.nacns.org/docs/CNSCoreCompetenciesBroch.pdf

Sparacino, P. S. A., & Cartwright, C. C. (2009). The clinical nurse specialist. In A. B. Hamric, J. A. Spross, & C. M. Hanson (Eds.), *Advanced practice nursing: An integrative approach* (pp. 349–379). St. Louis, MO: Saunders Elsevier.

CHAPTER 15

Reporting Out: Communicating to Multiple Audiences

MELANIE DUFFY
JANET S. FULTON

Clinical nurse specialist (CNS) practice is multifaceted, a fact well-substantiated in the literature. This multifaceted nature of CNS practice makes employing a CNS a great asset to an organization. The CNS is a go-to person with a broad and useful skill set. On the other hand, what makes a CNS such a valuable employee also makes the CNS a somewhat elusive employee. CNSs are keenly aware that the role is not well understood by nurses, other providers, administrators, and the public. In large part, the CNS role is not well understood because, well, nursing—what nursing practice is—is not well understood. CNSs, who practice nursing at an advanced level, are further challenged to explain. It's difficult to capture CNS practice and related outcomes in a succinct report. Feeling overwhelmed with where to start and bogged down by failure to create a perfect report, too many CNSs neglect to generate any reports. The increasing emphasis on accountability and outcomes demands that CNSs create, push forward, and develop some routine reports about their work efforts and related outcomes. This chapter offers suggestions for creating internal reports and ideas for disseminating professional practice initiatives externally.

TRACK YOUR WORK

Others don't understand CNS work because we have not always attended to the business of defining our work. CNSs impact the quality of care delivered in many ways, some highly visible such as leading by chairing quality committees, but many of our activities are more subtle, like modeling a best practice for a new nurse. Typically a CNS is involved in several projects or clinical initiatives at any one time. How should this work be defined in terms that could be put in a report? Linked to outcomes?

To report outcomes, begin by defining the work of your practice. Start writing down your daily activities. For example, if the day starts with making unit rounds, identify the "work" that occurs during those rounds—intervening with complex patients, supporting staff in implementing a new procedure, role-modeling interdisciplinary communication, checking equipment for safety concerns. Keep the list for a week. Organize the individual activities into groups. For example, general categories of activities might include: direct patient care activities; nurse/staff bedside education/coaching; formal educational programs; policy/procedure development; product review; evidence-based practice activities; quality monitoring. We will discuss more about categories later. Get a good sense of the work embedded in your CNS practice. Continue tracking your work intermittently—on 1 week, off 2 weeks—to get a good sample of your practice activities.

Next, list your job performance expectations. Performance expectations can come from multiple sources such as a job description, unit staff, management and administration, and other care providers. CNSs get pulled in a lot of directions; write down the expectations others have for you in the job. These expectations may include, for example, directives from administration, such as leading a falls prevention program, and informal expectations, such as a unit manager's request for assistance with roll out of a new cardiac monitoring procedure. Don't forget personal expectations. Addressing management priorities first is important for a new CNS in order to gain the confidence of coworkers and management. But keep personal expectations on the grid. Every CNS sees a gap between what is and what should be, and while it may not be possible to get to your agenda initially, the time will come.

Next step, reflect. Consider how the list of work activities will achieve the stated expectations. Make sure activities and performance expectations are aligned. Many a CNS struggles because activities and expectations are misaligned. Now align the expectations with the organization's mission and goals. Prioritize the expectations that most closely match the organization's mission, goals, and current priorities.

CREATE A WORKSHEET

Write the performance expectations as measurable objectives. For example, if you are expected to provide leadership for reducing catheter-associated urinary tract infections in the surgical population, write it as a measurable objective. Another expectation might be to mentor staff through the clinical ladder process, so write it as a measureable objective. Consider the practice activities (work) that need to be done to achieve the objectives. This exercise is extremely helpful in keeping CNS practice focused. Eliminate activities not directed at achieving targeted objectives. This exercise can help identify opportunities for maximizing time. For example, making daily unit rounds may be an excellent time to chat with staff nurses about the opportunities of the clinical ladder program while simultaneously uncovering any perceived barriers to the application procedure.

Create a grid for tracking progress toward achieving the objectives. Table 15.1 is an example of a tracking format that aligns practice activities with objectives. In the beginning it will be tedious and, yes, time consuming to break

TABLE 15.1 Example of a CNS Monthly Tracking Sheet

CNS Monthly Tracking	
Objectives	Activities/Progress
1. Reduce CAUTI to < 5% for surgical patients (6 South; 6 East; 5 South).	1.a. Implementing new protocol on indications for use of indwelling bladder catheters. 1.b. Conducting daily "catheter rounds" to ensure compliance/determine unintended consequences of new protocol.
2. Reduce cost of central line dressing kits with no increase in CLABSI.	2.a. Leading a task force. 2.b. Purpose, objectives, timeline, members established. 2.c. Samples of available kits obtained ($n = 6$). 2.d. Participating units identified: 2 East, 3 East, 3 South, 4 South. 2.e. Developing evaluation criteria.
3. Increase by 10 the number of successful clinical ladder applicants on surgical services (6 South; 6 East; 5 South).	3.a. Eight staff nurses attended information session/brown bag lunch (*date*). 3.b. Six nurses matched with "mentors." 3.c. Serving as mentor for two nurses. 3.d. Information session/brown bag scheduled for (*date*).

CAUTI, catheter-associated urinary tract infection; CLABSI, central line–associated bloodstream infection.

out the work at this micro level, but for the new CNS it is a useful way to make sure that work activities are aligned with measurable outcomes. It's also helpful for an experienced CNS who finds it difficult to achieve intended outcomes. Work and objectives can easily become misaligned. In naming practice activities (work), certain phrases will become common and used as shorthand for tracking. Select the best word to reflect an activity. For example, when the activity is to chair a committee or task force, use "leading" instead of "chairing" in the report. CNSs lead. Language is important. At the end of the year it will be possible to look down the list and summarize your "work" of a CNS. See Table 15.2 for a list of identified CNS functions (practice activities).

WHY A TRACKING SHEET?

What follows is a narrative of a CNS-led project to reduce catheter-associated urinary tract infection (CAUTI). While rich in detail, consider how it could be captured in a shorthand tracking sheet. How much of the narrative is about process? Are the outcomes evident? Are the outcomes quantified?

A CNS, as project coordinator, assembled a team to decrease the incidence of CAUTI. The infectious disease (ID) staff, clinical nursing staff, and physicians were invited to be members. Possible causes for the increase in infections were examined and included: (a) duration of urinary catheter use; (b) insertion/cleansing/discontinuation technique; (c) maintenance of an intact system; and (d) components of the insertion kit. The committee members agreed that all four components contributed to CAUTI.

The CNS and ID practitioners collaborated to develop a nurse-driven urinary catheter removal protocol based on current evidence. The protocol listed specific patient criteria to be met before an RN may remove a catheter. A CNS presented the protocol to the nursing/medical staff committees, staff informational/educational sessions were conducted, and the protocol was implemented.

Next, the CNS and ID practitioner made a video emphasizing the correct way to insert and discontinue indwelling urinary catheters. RN members of the committee, along with one or two nursing assistants, were recruited to participate in the video. The video was available to all clinical staff via computer system.

The CNS and ID representative made rounds on all nursing units to publicize the video, but more importantly, to discuss the adverse effects of prolonged catheter use and the importance of maintaining the integrity of the catheter system.

The CNS was also a member of the organization's Products and Equipment Committee. Contents of the urinary catheter insertion kit were examined and alternative kits were examined for ease of use.

Cost savings were calculated based on the difference in number of infections for the year before the change compared with the year after the change. The infection cost included additional days of hospitalization and additional medications/treatments. In addition, the number of urinary catheter kits used has decreased since fewer patients have indwelling urinary catheters. This cost savings can be attributed to the CNS.

In this example, CNS practice resulted in positive outcomes for patients and the organization. The CNS led the team and kept the project moving forward and on track. However, a narrative-reporting format makes it difficult to "see" the work of the CNS. You must first give language to your practice if you are to report on it. And a lengthy narrative will not get the attention of a busy administrator.

CREATE A SCORECARD

One reporting method is to use a scorecard (Muller, 2011). The CNS scorecard is a framework to measure the CNS's progress toward achievement of objectives and other organizational contributions. Scorecards can be personalized to fit performance expectations and may include, along with target objectives, measures of patient satisfaction scores, staff retention rates, journal club participation, and other metrics (Muller, 2011). Unlike a tracking sheet, a scorecard does not include activities, only outcomes.

In a comprehensive review of CNS practice outcomes, Doran, Sadani, and DiPietro (2014) identified specific activities illustrating direct and indirect practice functions by domain of practice (CNS sphere of influence). A summary of this work is in Table 15.2. The findings from this review of literature offer a possible framework for a scorecard. By using the categories of practice outcomes identified by Doran and colleagues, you would be creating an evidence-based scorecard. The patient care categories would include surveillance, provision of care, facilitation of support groups for patients and family, case management, and provision of consultation regarding patients' care. An educational category would include formal and informal educational functions. An organization-system category would be organized by continuous quality improvement initiatives, policies/procedures/best-practice guidelines development, program development and evaluation requiring intervention, evidence-based practice, and committee work. List your performance objectives under the categories and report measurable results.

TABLE 15.2 Direct and Indirect CNS Functions

Direct and Indirect Patient Care Functions

Direct Care	
Surveillance	1. Assessing patients' physical and psychosocial conditions, health behaviors and environmental situations 2. Diagnosing patient and family needs 3. Monitoring patients' conditions and progress toward achieving outcomes
Provision of care	1. Planning comprehensive care for patients and family 2. Providing extended education and counseling 3. Troubleshooting complex patient care problems 4. Assessing effectiveness of interventions
Facilitation of support groups for patients and family	1. Planning support groups for patients and family 2. Organizing logistics of support groups

(continued)

TABLE 15.2 Direct and Indirect CNS Functions (*continued*)

Direct and Indirect Patient Care Functions

Indirect Care	
Case management	1. Overseeing delivery of patient care 2. Facilitating interprofessional patient care conference 3. Conducting intra-/interprofessional services 4. Discharge planning, including arrangement for required community services
Provision of consultation regarding patients' care	1. Applying advanced knowledge in crisis intervention 2. Providing support for frontline problem solving, including equipment problems

Formal and Informal Education Functions

Formal	1. Participating in development, organization, and coordination of nursing staff orientation to specialty unit 2. Participating in initial and continuous assessment of nursing staff competencies 3. Designing and implementing ongoing educational programs for nursing staff based on identified learning needs/competencies 4. Providing certification renewal courses to nursing staff 5. Participating in and/or providing courses to undergraduate and/or graduate nursing students 6. Serving as a clinical preceptor to nursing staff and students
Informal	1. Providing mentorship to nursing staff at bedside 2. Serving as a role model in problem solving and case management 3. Serving as informal resource to nursing staff (e.g., responding to questions related to unfamiliar policies, procedures, clinical problems; discussing evidence base for nursing interventions)

(continued)

TABLE 15.2 Direct and Indirect CNS Functions (*continued*)

Direct and Indirect Patient Care Functions

Organization-System Domain of Practice Functions

Continuous quality improvement initiatives	1. Designing methods and tools for continuous collection of data (related to process and outcome of care) 2. Analyzing and synthesizing data obtained from multiple sources 3. Identifying care-related issues requiring remediation 4. Collaborating with members of intra-/interprofessional team in formulation of remedial strategies and change of practice 5. Overseeing implementation of remedial strategies and practice change 6. Facilitating ongoing outcome monitoring
Policies, procedures, and best-practice guidelines development	1. Developing organization policies and procedures related to care delivery 2. Developing best-practice guidelines based on available evidence 3. Providing leadership in dissemination and implementation of policies, procedures, and practice guidelines
Program development and evaluation requiring intervention	1. Collaborating with administrators and professionals (nursing and others) to identify clinical issues 2. Designing programs to address identified clinical issues 3. Coordinating implementation of programs and evaluation of their effects 4. Supporting nursing staff in change of practice or research utilization
Committee work	1. Participating in committees within the organization, community, and profession

CNS, clinical nurse specialist.
Source: Doran, Sidani, and DiPietro (2014). Reprinted with permission.

INTERNAL REPORTING OF OUTCOMES

Once the outcomes are captured, the next step is to figure out who needs to know what. Your direct line supervisor, aka "the boss," should receive a comprehensive report. This report is the basis of your annual performance review with the boss. Individual unit managers should receive snapshot reports about objectives relative to their assigned areas of responsibility. Administrators need summary reports demonstrating progress toward various system level goals and the organizational mission. Several short, customized reports are best. If the report must be more than one page, or include attachments such as tables, graphs or other information, be sure to have a brief summary page highlighting outcomes.

Don't wait to be asked to prepare and send reports. Just do it! A CNS once said she sent reports of quality-monitoring activities to the administrative team for almost a year before someone decided she should be invited to the quality committee because, as she explained, "they figured out I was doing work that was important to the organization."

EXTERNAL REPORTING OF PRACTICE INNOVATIONS

When achievement of outcomes includes innovative, cost-effective approaches to care, consider sharing the work with the larger professional community. Ask yourself if knowing how we achieved these outcomes would help someone else who likewise was striving for the same outcome. If the answer is yes, then disseminate your findings outside the organization. How? Prepare an abstract for presentation at a professional meeting or write an article for a professional journal, or both.

Start by identifying an appropriate professional meeting—a local, regional, or national nursing conference that has a call for abstracts. Professional meetings invite abstract submissions to ensure that their conferences have the latest, cutting-edge ideas. Find and review the call for abstracts—this is essentially the instructions for submitting. The call will include the topics of interest, format for the abstract, number of words for the title and body, the due date for submission, and any other specific instructions. Next, check employer procedures for submission of abstracts. Because the work was done as a part of your job, employers should give permission for the work to be submitted outside the organization. In most cases this is a formality, but check to make sure you are compliant with the "house rules" for dissemination. Also check with the internal (or institutional) review board (IRB) for protection of human subjects. Quality improvement projects are different from research studies; however, the IRB will make the final determination as to what can be disseminated outside of the organization. And of course, if the work was a research study, IRB approval would have been obtained *before* the study was conducted.

Complete the abstract following all the directions. The most common reason for an abstract to be rejected is because it did not comply with directions. Get help from a mentor if this is your first abstract. Have a colleague proofread the final draft. The second most common reason for rejection is poor grammar, misspelled words, missing content. Submit the abstract in the manner directed and on time. Abstracts received after the due date are not even reviewed. Once received, the abstract will be blind reviewed (also called "peer reviewed" or "juried"). It is sent to a panel of reviewers—they don't know the author, and the author doesn't know the panel members—where it is scored according to criteria. The criteria should have been included in the directions. Top-scoring abstracts are invited to present at the meeting.

Abstracts are presented as either posters or podium presentations. Posters are large (about 4 ft. x 6 ft.), one-page presentations with more in-depth information about the project than was in the abstract. Information on a poster usually includes the purpose, background, design, methods, outcomes, conclusions, and implications of the project. Posters are hung on large boards placed in rows at the conference where attendees can walk around, view the posters of interest, and discuss the work with the author who stands by the poster. Podium presentations are lecture-style presentations of the work, usually about 20 minutes long, and grouped in sessions with similar topics where three or four presentations take place one after the other.

Negotiate with the organization to pay all or part of any expenses involved in presenting at a professional meeting. But never, never, never stay home because the employer doesn't cover expenses. It's your career, and professional presentations are part of professional development. Be prepared to invest a portion of your salary in yourself.

It is quite prestigious to present your work at a professional meeting. Make sure this is a highlight of your reports!

ADDITIONAL READING

Charbachi, S., Williams, C., & McCormack, D. (2012). Articulating the role of the clinical nurse specialist in New Brunswick. *Nursing Leadership, 25*(2), 59–69.

Duffy, M., Daniels, K., Mittelstadt, P., & Muller, A. (2014). Impact of the clinical nurse specialist role on the costs and quality of healthcare. *Clinical Nurse Specialist, 28*(5), 300–303.

Finkelman, A. (2013). The clinical nurse specialist leadership in quality improvement. *Clinical Nurse Specialist, 27*(1), 31–35.

Fulton, J. (2013). Making outcomes of clinical nurse specialist practice visible. *Clinical Nurse Specialist, 27*(1), 5–6.

Jepsen, S. (2015). Using a scorecard to demonstrate clinical nurse specialists' contributions. *AACN Advanced Critical Care, 26*(1), 43–49.

Leary, A. (2011). How nurse specialists can demonstrate their worth. *Gastrointestinal Nursing, 9*(6), 46–49.

National Association of Clinical Nurse Specialists. (2004). *Statement on clinical nurse specialist practice and education.* Harrisburg, PA: NACNS.

Purvis, S., Brown, E., Chan, G., Dresser, S., Fulton, J., Koyama, K., & Tracy, M. F. (2012). The National Association of Clinical Nurse Specialists response to the Institute of Medicine's *The Future of Nursing* report. *Clinical Nurse Specialist, 26*(4), 222–224.

REFERENCES

Doran, D. M., Sidani, S., & DiPietro, T. (2014). Nurse-sensitive outcomes. In J. S. Fulton & K. A. Goudreau (Eds.), *Foundations of clinical nurse specialist practice*. New York, NY: Springer Publishing Company.

Muller, A., McCauley, K., Harrington, P., Jablonski, J., & Strauss, R. (2011). Evidence-based practice implementation strategy the central role of the clinical nurse specialist. *Nursing Administration Quarterly*, *35*(2), 140–151.

PART V
REACHING OUT

CHAPTER 16

Becoming Involved With Professional Organizations

MARY FRAN TRACY
PATRICK SCHULTZ

As you embark on a new career as a clinical nurse specialist (CNS), it may seem overwhelming to even consider getting involved in professional organizations. However, involvement in professional organizations can offer you a number of resource and networking opportunities and facilitate transition into your new role. Although active involvement may not be feasible right away, it is important to consider how simply being a member of a professional organization can benefit you as a new CNS. In addition, it may be helpful to keep in mind a target timeline for increasing professional involvement as a goal toward which to strive.

There can be many benefits of belonging to and being active in a professional organization. Getting involved in professional organizations as a CNS can offer both personal and professional rewards—professional self-development, networking and mentoring opportunities, development of advocacy skills, advancement of the profession of nursing, and ultimately improvement of patient care. With more than 80 (nursinglink.monster.com/education/articles/11850-the-ultimate-list-of-professional-associations-for-nurses) nursing organizations from which to choose, in addition to hundreds of additional multidisciplinary and specialty professional organizations, there are multiple options for finding an organization that matches your needs. This chapter gives you ideas to consider related to this aspect of your career path.

CHOOSING AN ORGANIZATION

If you were active in professional organizations prior to becoming a CNS, you may already be familiar with existing professional organizations. However, as a CNS student and novice CNS, you may now have different professional needs. This is a great time to explore other organizations. CNSs frequently belong to more than one professional organization. Organizations attract different members because they exist for different purposes. Some organizations are structured to meet the needs of nurses caring for certain patient populations, while some focus on nurses in certain roles. An organization may exist for a single profession, while other organizations are multidisciplinary (see Table 16.1).

What should you look for when you are deciding to join and become actively involved in a professional organization? Going to the organization's website can give you insight into the organization—its focus and priorities. Typically an organization will display its mission and vision on its website. Reviewing these statements should give you an overall view of the organization and its stated purpose for existing. Reviewing this information can give you a quick glimpse at the alignment of an organization with your goals and expectations as a member.

Reviewing other aspects of the organizational structure will give further insight into alignment: What are the organization's priorities? Do they match your expectations of how your dues would be spent? What is the leadership structure and how diverse are the leaders? Is it only a national organization,

TABLE 16.1 Examples of Professional Organizations

Organization Type	Website
Profession-Based Organizations	
American Nurses Association (ANA)	nursingworld.org
Constituent and State-Based ANA Organizations	nursingworld.org/affiliates.html
Multidisciplinary Organizations	
Society of Critical Care Medicine (SCCM)	www.sccm.org
American Heart Association (AHA)	www.heart.org/HEARTORG
American Diabetes Association (ADA)	www.diabetes.org
Role-Based Organizations	
National Association of Clinical Nurse Specialists (NACNS)	www.nacns.org
Association for Nursing Professional Development (ANPD)	www.anpd.org
American Organization of Nurse Executives (AONE)	www.aone.org
Population-Based Nursing Organizations	
American Association of Critical-Care Nurses (AACN)	www.aacn.org
Oncology Nursing Society (ONS)	www.ons.org
Wound, Ostomy, and Continence Nurses Society (WOCN)	www.wocn.org
American Psychiatric Nurses Association (APNA)	www.apna.org
Association of periOperative Registered Nurses (AORN)	www.aorn.org

Box 16.1   Potential Membership Benefits

- Journal subscriptions
- Newsletters
- Networking opportunities—internal and external to the organization
- "Representing your voice"
- Listserv participation
- Reduced rates for insurance or other group benefits
- Reduced rates for certification examinations
- Reduced registration fees to sponsored conferences
- Reduced rates for purchase of products
- Volunteer opportunities
- Continuing education opportunities
- Participation in a community of practice
- Promotion of and participation in research

or does it have a local, state, or regional structure as well? How long has the organization been in existence, and what are the demographics of its members? Exploring these questions can help you decide whether a particular organization meets your needs and expectations.

Websites may display a great deal of additional information and can be good resources, whether you actually join the organization as a member or simply use the resources in your CNS role. Many organizations post listings of educational offerings, organizational position statements, products for sale, and free resources on their web page. Websites will also typically list the cost of membership dues and the benefits that come with membership (see Box 16.1). While the actual amount of dues is a significant piece of information, it is also important to consider the monetary value of membership in context with the benefits—both tangible and intangible—of being a member.

BENEFITS OF PROFESSIONAL ORGANIZATION MEMBERSHIP AND INVOLVEMENT

Keeping Informed

A major benefit of membership is the opportunity for staying up to date in your area of specialty or interest. Many organizations publish journals or newsletters with the latest information. For a nursing organization with a clinical focus, journals frequently provide the latest practice developments and an opportunity to see how others are providing care for similar populations. Many organizations also provide content for continuing education in a variety of formats and fees. This is particularly important as you maintain requirements for your licensure and certifications. For organizations that are primarily role or profession focused, journals or newsletters may give updates on issues affecting your practice itself. Examples of this may include legislative activities that impact licensing or reimbursement, or activities impacting changes in professional standards.

Networking

Belonging to a professional organization is a great way to develop networks with colleagues who share your area of expertise or interest, both locally and across the country. Perhaps you are the only CNS in your specialty in your setting. Or perhaps you are, literally, the only CNS. Connecting with colleagues can reassure you that you are not alone in the challenges you are facing. It can connect you with colleague resources that you may not have known existed, even in your own immediate geographic area. Becoming involved can provide a reservoir of resources to tap into when needed. It can provide a mechanism to broaden your perspective and help you see solutions or opportunities that you may not have recognized or considered. These networking opportunities can present themselves through subscribing to member Listservs, networking at organizational conferences, and contacting organizational staff who can assist with helpful resources and contacts.

Connecting with colleagues can also offer insight into how other CNSs practice and how other CNS roles are structured. This can be valuable as you are developing in your own role and establishing your practice. Many new CNSs are interested in finding a mentor to help them as they begin their new career. Conversely, many experienced CNSs are committed to mentoring and fostering the development of novice CNSs. Involvement in an organization may help you find a colleague who would be a match as a mentor in the areas you are seeking to develop.

Opportunities for Professional Development

Activity in a professional organization can provide opportunities to develop leadership skills such as participating in and leading committees, helping groups come to consensus, and working on projects in a broader environment outside of work. Organizations are usually a mix of diverse members and perspectives. It is not uncommon when these diverse opinions lead to disagreements about actions or directions that should be taken. This creates an environment for you to develop and refine skills such as negotiation and conflict resolution, whether as an active member or as an organizational leader.

Many professional organizations are committed to providing education for their members. If you are interested in developing your presentation skills, you could offer to provide presentations at local or regional conferences. You may consider submitting abstracts for presentation at national conferences. You may also decide to develop your written communication skills by writing organizational newsletters or journals. Some organizations have created mentoring programs to partner nurses who are novices in these skills with more experienced nurses to copresent or coauthor.

Being a Role Model for Staff

An important role that should not be neglected is that of being an example for staff. A CNS's membership and involvement in professional organizations is a great role model for the staff members with whom the CNS works. Their involvement as members or certificants will give them benefits similar to yours. The successful CNS is one who enables staff members to independently look at evidence for best practice. Membership can provide staff members with resources that are evidence-based and can support them in critically evaluating their practice. In addition, your role modeling helps create enthusiasm and cohesiveness as a profession. A deeper collegial relationship is often formed among members of the same organization.

Contributing to the Profession

Belonging to and being active in professional organizations benefits not only you but benefits also the profession of nursing. Organizations advance the profession of nursing by generating and capitalizing on financial power, political power, and intellectual power through their membership. Your membership dues help generate financial power, which allows for strategic investments. These strategic investments can include research funds to advance the science of nursing and improve patient care, political investments that can impact advancements in the profession that affect your practice, and investments in nurses that can offer access to professional growth opportunities.

Political power is generated by unifying nurses throughout districts, states, regions, countries, and the world. As membership grows, so does the ability to influence legislators and stakeholders. Organizations develop positions based on the views of their members. As an active member you can use your professional organization to influence patient care and the nursing profession by making your views known. The organization has the strength and cohesiveness to augment the voices of members through advocacy and structure. In addition, as a member you may be able to take advantage of organizational resources for developing your own personal advocacy skills. Organizations have the resources to effect change that individual professionals may not be able to accomplish.

Intellectual power is generated by the coming together of diverse perspectives in nursing. Combining the thoughts of leaders from differing backgrounds, interests, and educational fields can create formal or informal think tanks where unique solutions to problems and ideas for research and practice innovations can be generated. Having many perspectives can contribute to achieving goals as a group, whereas an individual working alone might not have such success. As a member, you benefit from facilitated access to these diverse colleagues.

The presence of nursing is established by the activities of professional organizations. They gather the attention of thè media and the public. This is an important way for people to find out who nurses really are and what they really do. Stereotypes can be dismantled. Many organizations provide resources that you can use in your daily role to educate the public about what nurses and CNSs do. By attending meetings and networking with colleagues, you can showcase the CNS role to other nurses and professionals.

Professional nursing organizations give nurses the opportunity to stand alongside other professional organizations, thereby ensuring the nursing perspective is heard. By using your voice through your professional organization, you are influencing patient care and the nursing profession. Since membership organizations rely on knowing and meeting member needs, your needs can be addressed at the same time the needs of the nursing profession are addressed.

Getting Started

At this point, you hopefully realize the benefits for you and nursing by your being involved in a professional organization. The first steps to investigating professional organizations to join may be triggered by a variety of reasons. As a CNS student looking toward graduation, exploring organizations that offer certification may be your first priority in connecting with an organization. Frequently, members of an affiliated organization pay a reduced fee to take the certification exam. As a new CNS, having access to journals and newsletters may be important. A frequent benefit of membership is receipt of organizational publications and may even include reduced or free access to online evidence-based resources not available to nonmembers or the general public. Knowing which journals and newsletters are important to your professional practice guides you to the organizations that publish those resources. As mentioned previously, reviewing organizational information online will quickly give you perspective on what activities the organization is involved in and how the organization focuses its priorities. Attending either local or national conferences will give you a good sense of the organization, its fit for you, and opportunities for networking.

It may be easier to start organizational involvement at the local level. The organization's website will typically provide contact information on local, state, or regional chapters, offices, and websites. It is important to establish whether membership at a local level also requires membership at a national level. Find out the local meeting schedule and whether you need to be a member to attend or if you can attend either as a guest or for a fee. If you know a colleague who is a member, ask if you can attend an event to get to know the organization. It's easier to go with someone you know.

Volunteering

Once you decide to join an organization, don't be surprised if you are approached to volunteer for the organization. Resist the urge to assume you don't have the necessary skills to be a volunteer leader. Consider how volunteering will fit within your professional and personal lives. There are many ways to volunteer, and most organizations are willing to negotiate and utilize whatever time and skills you are able to offer. Consider offering to volunteer in ways that fit your time and lifestyle commitments. If you have a particular skill, it may be convenient to offer that skill in volunteering. Conversely, if you are looking to develop new skills and have the time to devote to that development, consider volunteering in an area that will be new and challenging for you with adequate support for development.

Most organizations have a variety of volunteer opportunities that can match your availability for time commitment. Don't hesitate to be clear about what you are able to offer in terms of time and commitment to ensure there is a match. Volunteer opportunities come in many different forms—from joining committees with face-to-face meetings, to performing volunteer work from home, to participating in a conference call to provide ideas or feedback. If you are interested in volunteering at the national level, most organizations will post a call for volunteers through their newsletters or websites. They may also maintain a member volunteer database, which is queried by the organization when a particular interest, skill, or volunteer commitment is needed. Regardless of how you choose to volunteer, carefully consider what you are committing to in order to avoid the unfortunate circumstance of having to withdraw at a later date due to an inability to fulfill the commitment. Foremost, enjoy your volunteerism as an opportunity to broaden your horizons and acquire new collegial relationships that will enrich your professional career.

SUMMARY

Inevitably you will be attracted to many different organizations for various personal reasons. Choosing the actual number of professional organizations you will join and in which you become an active member should be a thoughtful process. This process should include consideration of priorities, choosing an organization, and determining the level of involvement.

First, evaluate your priority needs and interests. These priorities will help you determine whether to choose a specialty population-related organization, a role-based organization, a multidisciplinary organization, or a profession-based organization. From those priorities, explore your options and choose one or more organizations to join.

Then, determine your level of involvement. Keep your purpose for joining clearly in mind. As a novice CNS, be careful not to overextend yourself. A balance must be found between expending energy to become proficient in your new role and taking on more responsibility within professional organizations. However, the novice CNS must also be careful not to automatically say no to all new opportunities. It can be easy to think there is no time to become involved in the important work of professional organizations.

Finally, take time to evaluate how well your time and energy are being managed. Are you getting what you need out of your memberships? Are you able to honor your commitments adequately? As you develop in your role, you will continue to gain new perspectives about your professional needs, anticipating they will change over the course of your career. This may result in changes or additions to affiliations over time.

Transitioning to the CNS role can itself be challenging, and it can be easy to defer joining and becoming an active member of professional organizations. However, becoming an active member of just one professional organization can provide innumerable opportunities for networking, professional development, and access to resources, which can be invaluable as a new CNS.

ADDITIONAL READING

Haylock, P. J. (2013). Professional nursing organizations: Meeting needs of nurses and the profession. In D. J. Mason, J. K. Leavitt, & M. W. Chaffee (Eds.), *Policy and politics in nursing and health care* (6th ed., pp. 609–617). St. Louis, MO: Saunders.

Mata, H., Latham, T. P., & Ransome, Y. (2010). Benefits of professional organization membership and participation in national conferences: Considerations for students and new professionals. *Health Promotion Practice, 11*(4), 450–453.

Schroeder, R. T. (2013). The value of belonging to a professional nursing organization. *AORN Journal, 98*(2), 99–101. doi:10.1016/j.aorn.2013.06.002

Shinn, L. (2013). Current issues in nursing associations. In D. J. Mason, J. K. Leavitt, & M. W. Chaffee (Eds.), *Policy and politics in nursing and health care* (6th ed., pp. 602–608). St. Louis, MO: Saunders.

Spratt, D. (2012). Collaborating to give back to our professional organization. *AORN Journal, 96*(6), 567–569. doi:10.1016/j.aorn.2012.10.012

Tracy, M. F., & Hanson, C. M. (2013). Leadership. In A. B. Hamric, C. M. Hanson, M. F. Tracy, & E. T. O'Grady (Eds.), *Advanced practice nursing: An integrative approach* (5th ed., pp. 266–298). St. Louis, MO: Saunders.

Wilson, C. (2014). Return on investment for professional organization membership. *Journal for Nurses in Professional Development, 30*(4), 215–216. doi:10.1097/NND.0000000000000091

CHAPTER 17

Working With Community Agencies

SHARON D. HORNER
CARA C. YOUNG
KAREN E. JOHNSON

Despite improvements in some areas of health over the past century (e.g., reductions in infectious disease, increased life expectancy), advances in technology to treat disease, and the fact that we spend substantially more money on health care than any other nation, America continues to lag behind other developed countries—and sees great disparities within our borders—in crucial health indicators such as obesity, diabetes, heart disease, low birth weight, and teen pregnancy (National Research Council and Institute of Medicine, 2013). Patients admitted to hospitals today have higher acuities, require more complex care, and are discharged earlier than in previous decades. Further, they must learn how to manage their complex care at a time when they are feeling fatigued and dealing with symptoms (Logue & Drago, 2013). As a result, postdischarge care is fraught with errors due to communication problems, low health literacy, and fragmentation of care that have contributed to high hospital readmission rates. In response, the Affordable Care Act of 2010 imposed a penalty for hospital readmissions within 30 days for select conditions (Logue & Drago, 2013). But the Affordable Care Act also established the Community-Based Care Transitions Program with funding to support health systems and community-based organizations in working together to provide transitional services to high-risk Medicare beneficiaries (Naylor, Aiken, Kurtzman, Olds, & Hirschmann, 2011). The clinical nurse specialist (CNS) is in an ideal position to lead these transition care programs and to establish collaborations between acute care, chronic care, public health and community-based organizations as ways are sought to improve the health of the clients served as well as the greater community. The focus of this chapter is on building collaborations and working with community agencies to extend the CNS's spheres of influence.

Community Agencies

Community agencies include entities that focus on physical health, emotional health, social health, and environmental health, as well as those that do not have an explicit focus on health. Organizations/agencies may serve geographic communities or communities that share identities based on culture, health conditions, faith, race/ethnicity, or institutions. Traditionally, CNSs have had few, if any, opportunities to work with smaller community health-related agencies and non-health-related community agencies during formal graduate school. However, changes to the health care landscape—including the downsizing of hospitals and movement of care into the community—will require CNSs to become competent and comfortable navigating the complex network of community agencies that serve clients where they live, work, and play (Patten & Goudreau, 2012). Benefits of community collaboration can accrue to patients, to the community, to the institution that employs the CNS, and to the CNS.

BENEFITS TO PATIENTS

CNS practice is designed to improve patient-focused outcomes (Patten & Goudreau, 2012). In collaboration with community agencies, the CNS can address health issues in the community that have the potential to improve patients' quality of life. Collaborative activities vary according to unique community needs but may include such activities as working with public health nurses and other community-based professionals to conduct community assessments, plan community-based health programs, create resource banks (e.g., lending libraries, mobility aids, food pantries) for community members, and testifying before health or governmental boards or committees. When health interventions are conceptualized on a continuum that ranges from primary prevention strategies (e.g., flu shots, in-home safety assessments for fall prevention) to clinical therapeutic measures (e.g., screening, rehabilitation, palliation), then community outreach can be seen as a natural extension of CNS practice (Baldwin, Black, & Hammond, 2014).

BENEFITS TO THE COMMUNITY

Effective strategies that address health needs and reduce health disparities within communities require collaboration among individuals, groups, and organizations. Community-based health programs need to address the environmental (e.g., parks, sidewalks), social (e.g., social isolation), political (e.g., willingness to invest in prevention), and economic (e.g., poverty) factors that influence health care and health promotion activities (Israel, Eng, Schulz, & Parker, 2013).

A simple Google search yields a variety of community coalitions that have evolved to meet diverse community needs. Coalitions have been established at the local, regional, statewide, and national levels to streamline fundraising activities for nonprofit organizations, balance economic growth while protecting the environment, raise the quality of life in a neighborhood or town, as well as targeting single issues such as long-term care, family violence, or networking with politicians (Israel et al., 2013). Many larger towns and cities have health-related coalitions that serve as mechanisms for the different, and sometimes competing, institutions to meet and work together on solving community-wide problems. For example, the Maternal, Child, and Family Health Coalition of Metropolitan St. Louis brings together over 200 agencies to promote healthy families to collectively address women's health care, prenatal care, maternal mental health, immunizations, and healthy home environments. When the CNS reaches out to community agencies, institutional and community agency resources can be leveraged to reach underserved populations or to tackle more complex health issues than individual organizations could accomplish independently.

BENEFITS TO THE INSTITUTION

The CNS's expertise is a valuable asset of the institution. The mandate to reduce costly 30-day hospital readmissions can be viewed as a major driving force for changing the model of care delivery (Naylor et al., 2011). Sustainable transition care programs should build on existing resources both within and outside of the acute care hospital system. Community-based organizations can provide vital supportive services that can help discharged patients make a successful transition to home or extended care (Baldwin et al., 2014). In fact, establishing collaborations with community-based organizations for coordination of care can benefit the institution as it works with community partners to build successful, sustainable transition care networks that together will improve patient outcomes and reduce costs associated with preventable 30-day readmissions (Naylor et al., 2011).

BENEFITS TO THE CNS

Finally, the CNS can derive both professional and personal benefits by working with community agencies. Over time, as the CNS's expertise is recognized outside the institution, opportunities to contribute to a wide range of health-related issues will emerge. In turn, the CNS gains a sense of personal satisfaction as quality improvements are made available in the greater community. Finally, the CNS can derive both professional and personal benefits by working with community-based organizations to improve the health of the community (Patten & Goudreau, 2012). By helping to establish and maintain collaborations with community-based organizations, the CNS will begin to be recognized as a valued colleague by the community and an important asset for the institution (Baldwin et al., 2014).

Getting Started

The CNS should have a goal in mind when setting out to build connections with community agencies. Having a goal can help focus the CNS in identifying, contacting, and working with community agencies. For CNSs who are novices or experienced CNSs who are new to a community, the goal may simply be to identify the community resources available for a selected population and then to volunteer in community organizations that provide resources or services that are applicable to that population (Israel et al., 2013). Volunteering serves to introduce the CNS to community groups and is one means of building social capital. For established CNSs who have or who are developing programs of care for a selected population, the goal would most likely be focused on ways to extend the program of care into the community (Baldwin et al., 2014). A few examples of broadly defined community-based goals include reducing chronic diseases, increasing and facilitating access to health and social services, improving the quality of life of persons with chronic conditions, or preventing injury and illness.

TABLE 17.1 Reaching Out to Community Agencies: Getting Started

1. Identify community agencies
   Agencies that provide health care services or resources:
   Hospitals
   Clinics
   Health department (state, local)
   Hospice
   Medical supply vendors
   Emergency medical services
   Funeral/mortuary vendors
   Pharmaceutical companies (e.g., drug assistance programs)
   Organizations/groups with primary focus on health care:
   Professional associations
   Support groups (in-person and virtual)
   School nurses
   Parish nurses
   Other community agencies:
   Churches, synagogues, temples
   Schools, colleges, universities
   Parks and leisure programs
   Library
   Exercise facilities
   Transportation vendors
   Legal services, law enforcement
   Businesses
   Community action agencies
   Day care

(continued)

TABLE 17.1 Reaching Out to Community Agencies: Getting Started (*continued*)

1. Identify community agencies (*continued*)
Food pantries Disaster preparedness organizations (e.g., the Red Cross) Homeowners associations/neighborhood associations City council
2. Contact community agencies
Cold call/e-mail/in-person visit Volunteer services, general Volunteer to serve on specific project (e.g., community assessment) Search for collaborative projects Propose collaborative projects
3. Work with community agencies
Develop relationships Define issues to address (e.g., community assessment) Plan a community-based health intervention Implement the intervention Evaluate the intervention
4. Maintain collaborative relationships
Invest time to maintain relationships Facilitate entry of colleagues into organization

IDENTIFYING COMMUNITY AGENCIES

Community health promotion interventions can be implemented by organized systems (e.g., community agencies, coalitions) or driven by grass roots efforts (e.g., neighborhood groups, community "watch dog" groups). The CNS begins by identifying community agencies or coalitions the mission or functional activities of which are congruent with the goal selected. For example, if the goal is to improve the quality of life for persons with a selected chronic condition, the CNS would identify agencies that serve the selected population including formal organizations (e.g., American Heart Association, American Lung Association, American Cancer Society), and health care–based resources (e.g., Breast Cancer Support Group, Camp for All). However, the CNS should also look beyond these agencies to identify other groups or agencies that have the potential to contribute to quality of life in the realm of social or emotional functioning (Israel et al., 2013). For example, the community library may sponsor book clubs for groups with different interests, or a local specialty school (e.g., culinary or art school) might provide community classes that could be tailored to meet the needs of special groups.

The inclusion of non-health-related agencies into a comprehensive health promotion initiative has the potential to yield important benefits to patients and the community partners.

CONTACTING COMMUNITY AGENCIES

The CNS begins by gaining entrée into these community agencies (Israel et al., 2013). Public agencies have newsletters or websites that explain missions, scopes of practice, and lists of meetings and activities. The CNS can attend open meetings to learn more about the agency and to meet agency representatives. Because of their collaborative structure, community coalitions have meetings that are open to the community that would be an easy point of entry for the CNS.

When the agency does not have open meetings, the CNS needs to establish entrée to the agency. Connections can be established through networking with colleagues, or by simply reaching out cold to agencies via a combination of phone calls, e-mails, and in-person appearances at the agency. Reaching out in person can be particularly effective, as people who receive numerous e-mails and phone calls each day might overlook an e-mail from a stranger. Networking can begin in the workplace as the CNS discusses his or her goals for community collaborations over lunch or before other institutional meetings. Established colleagues will offer advice and may have contacts with community agencies. Colleagues' introductions to community agency personnel can ease the CNS's entry into the agencies (Ansmann et al., 2014). The CNS also needs to attend professional meetings in the community to build collegial relationships outside the workplace because representatives of community agencies may attend these local meetings. Such informal networking is a good way to begin reaching out to community agencies, and similarly the CNS should not overlook the value of volunteering his or her services to support the agency's projects as a means of establishing connections with community agencies (Ansmann et al., 2014).

It is important to note that successful community partnerships are true collaborations that incorporate the expertise of all partners—not just the expertise of those with the most advanced degrees. In a clinic/hospital setting, the CNS may be used to being looked to as the "expert" on how to address health issues. When moving into the community, the CNS must go humbly, recognizing that both his or her expertise as well as the expertise brought by community partners and residents will be needed in order to adequately meet the needs of clients.

WORKING WITH COMMUNITY AGENCIES

Successfully working with a community agency to improve the health of individuals within the community the CNS mutually serve requires an understanding and appreciation of the mission, goals, and structure of the community partner. Community agencies have professional staff, nonprofessional support staff, and volunteers who work together to achieve the agency's mission and goals. This diverse mix of expertise and experience can be challenging when working with community agencies. At the same time, innovative and creative solutions can result from the synergy experienced as the group explores diverse ways of conceptualizing issues and different approaches to the same problem. It is essential to acknowledge that the inherent values and goals of an organization will influence the ways in which they wish to approach improving health within the community. Perhaps the most important rule is to *keep an open mind* when working with community agencies, recognizing that there are many different approaches that can be taken when developing and implementing health promotion initiatives (Israel et al., 2013). The major activities to accomplish an effective partnership include: (a) building relationships with community agencies, (b) defining issues to address, (c) planning community-based health interventions, and (d) implementing and evaluating the health promotion intervention.

Developing Relationships With Community Agencies

Developing and sustaining collaborative relationships with community partners is a fundamental component of community-based health promotion programs; it is also considered one of the most challenging components of successful programming (Israel et al., 2013). Adequate time should be devoted before the initiation of any community-based project to interagency infrastructure development including establishment of a leadership structure involving relevant organizational and community stakeholders. The nature of the collaborative structure, mission, and decision-making processes should be established (Yoo et al., 2003). It takes time to develop this infrastructure as the partners will need to consider the different imperatives under which their agencies function in order to arrive at workable processes for collaboration (Yoo et al., 2003). The work to establish infrastructure does not take place in isolation; rather, it will emerge as agency representatives define the issues to address and prioritize activities. Inevitably organizational restrictions (e.g., policy, mission) or legal imperatives (e.g., Health Insurance Portability and Accountability Act [HIPAA], Family Educational Rights and Privacy Act [FERPA]) under which the collaborating partners operate will be identified and must be taken into consideration in the planning process. Relationship building is an ongoing process throughout collaboration and should continue to evolve even after a project is completed. In the spirit of coalition building, the CNS should also look for opportunities to connect organizations with each other.

Defining Issues to Address

When working with community agencies to design health promotion initiatives, it is important for the partners to agree upon the goal or endpoint toward which they are working. As issues are discussed, it may become advantageous to expand the partnership to include community representatives from the target population in the form of a community advisory board (e.g., specific ethnic groups or selected health conditions), government officials or neighborhood representatives, and other community agencies or organizations

(Lian, Kohler, & Ross, 2015). The potential contribution of an additional partner should be considered in terms of the resources and perspectives each may bring to improve the partnership's ability to effectively define and address a community health problem (Lian et al., 2015).

Gathering data about the community can facilitate the partner's work to identify salient issues and create goals. Community assessments should include describing how the community is defined and organized, recognizing key stakeholders, and identifying assets and resources as well as barriers and issues of concern (Israel et al., 2013). If previous community programs have attempted to address health issues in the past, assessment of the strengths, weaknesses, level of community involvement, and the degree of success achieved with each program may provide valuable insight into the current initiative. Inevitably more issues will be identified than can be addressed in one intervention or project. Issues may be prioritized based on a number of criteria including the time-sensitive nature of the issue, available resources for addressing the issue, complexity of the issue, and severity of the issue. A wise strategy for new collaborators to follow would be to select an issue that is manageable in scope, fits the available resources (both financial and nonfinancial), and has a good potential for success. Success with smaller projects can serve as the impetus to tackle more complex projects.

Planning Community-Based Health Interventions

Once the team has been established, an issue selected, and goals defined, the process of intervention planning must be undertaken. Bartholomew, Parcel, Kok, Gottlieb, and Fernandez (2011) suggest intervention planning (i.e., development of an action plan) includes two primary steps: (a) identification of theory-based intervention methods and practical applications, and (b) development of the intervention program. During these steps, program ideas are discussed and selected based on theoretical and practical considerations; application methods are identified; and intervention components are drafted, pretested (if feasible), modified based on initial feedback, and implemented (Bartholomew et al., 2011). An important part of the planning phase is involvement of representatives from the target population. Ensuring adequate representation of the intended audience during the planning phase improves the chances of acceptability to the end user and may help identify early certain barriers to successful implementation (Israel et al., 2013). Depending on the nature of the program and established partnership, this might mean involvement of the community members already invested in the partnership or recruitment of additional representatives.

As the partners create and refine the interventions, they will need to determine the type and quantity of resources needed to implement the plan. Financial support is needed for some but not all of the tasks. Some resources may be provided by the partners such as meeting space, duplication services, news items or ads in newsletters or flyers that are routinely produced by the agency, volunteers, and clerical support (Israel et al., 2013). No-cost resources should also be sought such as free advertising through public service announcements on local television and radio stations and the educational materials available from national health-based organizations. Other resources may require funding and therefore a task force may be organized to develop and submit proposals to foundations or other charitable organizations seeking grants to support the project.

Implementing the Intervention

The action plan will guide the implementation of the intervention. Effective health promotion interventions include process and summative evaluations. The action plan should include procedures for obtaining feedback from both the consumers and the interveners during implementation and after the intervention is completed (Bartholomew et al., 2011). Community partners and members of the planning committee need to use the process evaluation data to identify and correct problems during implementation. This process includes creating methods for data collection, determining which components of participant feedback to address, and deciding how to approach integrating the changes into the intervention (Israel et al., 2013). The partnership should also attempt to anticipate potential challenges and barriers to implementation prior to initiation in order to respond more effectively as issues inevitably arise. Some questions to consider might be: How will the methods be modified if community participation is lacking? How will the fidelity of the intervention across sites be ensured? What strategies could be initiated to ensure adequate time to carry out intervention activities?

Evaluating the Intervention

Fundamental within the process of intervention planning, implementation, and evaluation is the assumption that the knowledge gained during each prior phase (i.e., assessment, planning, implementation, and evaluation) leads directly to the next step. As experience and knowledge of the evaluative process is gained, the partners can move back and forth between steps (Bartholomew et al., 2011). Therefore, evaluation is an ongoing activity throughout implementation of the program and should include feedback on the process, the program itself, and ideally health or quality of life outcomes that provide evidence for the effectiveness of the intervention.

Summative evaluation of the intervention should include assessment of program satisfaction as well as measurement of the selected health or health-related outcomes. Other indirect factors could also be assessed such as level of awareness and knowledge of the health issue, resources available to assist with the health issue, or willingness of community members to consider implementing certain health behaviors. While assessing the success of the intervention is important, the extent to which the clinician–community partnership is successfully collaborating to address improvement of health in the community must also be critically evaluated (Israel et al., 2013). Undertaking a process of self-reflection and critical appraisal will give members of the partnership an opportunity to voice their experiences and highlight areas in need of strengthening.

MAINTAINING COLLABORATIVE RELATIONSHIPS

Establishing collaborative relationships with community agencies, while challenging, is well worth the CNS's investment. The CNS needs to continue investing time and effort in maintaining these relationships. As noted earlier, success in implementing health promotion projects can lead to further and potentially more comprehensive collaborations that have the potential to benefit the greater community. Having established a working relationship with community agencies, the CNS may then be able to facilitate the entrée of colleagues into community agencies to further serve the greater community. Factors that were found to be critical to successful community-based collaborative health interventions included:

- Identifying an important unmet need
- Having people with the necessary skills, expertise, and commitment see the project through to completion
- Paying careful attention to the planning process
- Having good collaboration between the partners
- Having an inclusive leadership style
- Maintaining a clear focus on the targeted consumers of the program (Bartholomew et al., 2011; Israel et al., 2013; Lian et al., 2015)

SUMMARY

Reaching out to community agencies is a vital option for building a community's capacity to effectively improve the health of the community. Given the current shift toward transitional care with increasing emphasis on community-based services, this is an ideal time for the CNS to build collaborative relationships with community partners to improve the health of the community in which he or she practices.

REFERENCES

Ansmann, L., Flickinger, T. E., Barello, S., Kunneman, M., Mantwill, S., Quilligan, S., ... Aelbrecht, K. (2014). Career development for early career academics: Benefits of networking and the role of professional societies. *Patient Education and Counseling, 97,* 132–134.

Baldwin, K. M., Black, D., & Hammon, S. (2014). Developing a rural transitional care community case management program using clinical nurse specialists. *Clinical Nurse Specialist, 28,* 147–155.

Bartholomew, L. K., Parcel, G. S., Kok, G., Gottlieb, N. H., & Fernandez, M. E. (2011). *Planning health promotion programs* (3rd ed.). San Francisco, CA: Jossey-Bass.

Israel, B. A., Eng, E., Schulz, A. J., & Parker, E. A. (2013). *Methods for community-based participatory research for health* (2nd ed.). Hoboken, NJ: John Wiley & Sons.

Lian, B., Kohler, C. L., & Ross, L. (2015). On some practical considerations regarding community participatory research for addressing cancer health disparities. *Journal of Cancer Education, 30.* Retrieved from http://link.springer.com.ezproxy.lib.utexas.edu/article/10.1007/s13187-014-0782-z

Logue, M. D., & Drago, J. (2013). Evaluation of a modified community-based care transitions model to reduce costs and improve outcomes. *BMC Geriatrics, 13,* 94. Retrieved from http://www.biomedcentral.com/1471-2318/13/94

National Research Council and Institute of Medicine. (2013). Shorter lives, poorer health. In S. H. Woolf & L. Aron (Eds.), *U.S. health in international perspective.* Washington, DC: The National Academies Press.

Naylor, M. D., Aiken, L. H., Kurtzman, E. T., Olds, D. M., & Hirschman, K. B. (2011). The importance of transitional care in achieving health reform. *Health Affairs, 30,* 746–754.

Patten, S., & Goudreau, K. A. (2012). The bright future for clinical nurse specialist practice. *Nursing Clinics of North America, 47,* 193–203.

Yoo, S., Shada, R. E., Goodman, R. M., Weed, N. E., Lempa, M. L., & Mbondo, M. (2003). Collaborative community empowerment: An illustration of a six-step process. *Health Promotion Practice, 4,* 1–10.

CHAPTER 18

Networking

MARY A. STAHL

Networking is a valuable activity in any profession. The clinical nurse specialist (CNS) will find that networking can expedite and add value to contributions in the workplace, stimulate new ideas and approaches to problems, provide opportunities for professional skill development and awareness of career opportunities, and increase personal satisfaction. This chapter describes networking on a variety of levels, starting within the employment setting, then in the local community, and finally on a broader scale. A variety of examples are identified to provide ideas on how to access these networks and the types of opportunities they provide.

What is networking? According to the organization Women Into the Network, networking is simply "connecting with people of like interests and uncovering opportunities" (n.d.). Networking is forming relationships with other people to learn and grow from the reciprocal exchange of ideas, advice, and experiences (Scott, 2007). While communicating with people we know is an everyday activity, the purposeful approach of establishing contacts for networking may feel uncomfortable to some. The benefits, however, are well worth the effort.

Basically you are getting to know people and they are getting to know you. Be open, friendly, and an astute listener. Have a question in mind as an ice-breaker that relates to the situation where you are meeting others, and show a genuine interest in learning about them. If you are new to a work setting, the question "What brought you to work here?" will generally get people talking and may give you useful information about your employer. Asking others about their work—or if outside your work setting, their thoughts on a speaker or conference you are both attending—may be an easy way to open a conversation. Be comfortable talking about yourself both professionally and personally, and be sure to ask questions to learn more about the other person.

To increase your comfort and success with networking, prepare. Dialoguing with someone you've just met is as much about learning as about sharing, and can challenge you to think quickly. Be aware of current events, professional issues and trends, and think through a position on these topics so you will have something meaningful to say. There is no need to dominate the conversation;

contribute, be interesting or thought-provoking, and you will be memorable to others.

If there is an opportunity to provide information or a resource that is of interest to the other person, do so as long as this doesn't disclose information that is confidential to your employer. Some employers consider protocols, order sets, and the like to be proprietary and will not want you sharing with organizations that they consider to be competitors. Sharing resources when possible and sharing experiences and ideas help form a positive impression that will aid in developing at least a contact or perhaps a relationship. To dispel a misconception from the business community, the goal is the relationship, not identifying what the other person can do for you.

NETWORKING WITHIN YOUR HOSPITAL OR SYSTEM

When starting a new position, some initial contacts, such as your immediate supervisor or the person assigned to help with orientation to the institution and role, will be identified for you. Others will become apparent in your clinical area, such as the clinical and formal leaders and the interdisciplinary team members. Relationships with physicians and other professionals most frequently encountered in your practice area are well worth cultivating so that practice issues and change projects will be easier to negotiate when they arise. The nursing staff will help you understand the processes, both formal and informal, that frame the work they do every day. Their insights will help you understand what is working and what is not working, and will identify the challenges and work-arounds that occur on a routine basis. This will help you understand where to focus your efforts to make the most meaningful contributions to patient safety, clinical excellence, evidence-based practice, and unit culture. Key relationships to develop will include the CNSs and other advanced practice registered nurses (APRNs) within the hospital and system. They will be invaluable in helping you understand the ways in which APRNs have had impact in the organization, and will have insight into the formal and informal approval processes. If your hospital is part of a health care system, developing relationships in other system entities can be valuable, particularly in the clinical areas most similar to your practice.

Be alert to opportunities to develop relationships throughout the organization. Participation in various projects and workgroups may bring contact with administrators, a quality analyst, the person who negotiates insurance reimbursement contracts, purchasing, or the legal department, among others. Volunteering for projects with broad impact is a great way to get to know people, demonstrate your skills, and develop relationships. These are unique opportunities to network, not only putting a face with a name, but creating an impression so that when you reach out with a question or request, the person is likely to remember you.

The relationships developed within your work environment will be crucial in day-to-day activities and in your ability to create change. These individuals can contribute different perspectives to help fully analyze an issue and evaluate potential solutions. They will include key leaders whose support will move projects forward and can provide insight to address barriers. Some will be able to provide a broader view of the organization and other initiatives that are occurring, which will be valuable information as you anticipate challenges and opportunities for your practice area and for your involvement at the institutional or system level.

NETWORKING WITHIN YOUR LOCAL COMMUNITY

Developing relationships beyond your institution in your local community also brings value. Seek groups with like interests, such as CNS or APRN groups, local chapters of national clinical specialty groups, or Sigma Theta Tau chapters (see Chapter 15). Individuals you meet through these groups will have interests in common with you. Find opportunities to make connections within local academic institutions. Local continuing education programs provide the opportunity to meet colleagues from other hospitals in your area. Become active in voluntary health agencies, volunteering your time and expertise. Even participation in community or civic groups may yield networking chances; take the opportunity to get to know people through your faith organization, children's school, or at the dog park or community events.

These networking opportunities may provide an expanded view of your institution within the community. If you are considering changing positions, you may learn of job opportunities or have the chance to learn about other employers in ways that do not come through in an interview. Viewpoints from outside your organization may help bring new perspectives on issues you are addressing or new ideas for solutions. You may find mentors or the opportunity to collaborate on projects that benefit multiple hospitals, such as a stroke education consortium, multisite research, or performance-improvement project (Kleinpell & Hravnak, 2005). If you are working with a program that reaches into the community for health screening and promotion or education, contacts within community organizations may facilitate access to target populations or help refine your approach.

NETWORKING ON A BROADER SCALE

With the skills and confidence you have developed through networking in your local area, you are now ready to expand your network to a national or even international level. Attending a national conference provides numerous opportunities to network: in the registration line, lunch line, or as you wait for a session to begin. Take advantage of social opportunities and events that are created for just this purpose. Easy icebreakers may be "Where do you work?" or a comment on one of the speakers or sessions you have enjoyed. Some conferences recruit attendees to introduce speakers. This can be an opportunity to meet someone you admire or who has done work on a topic in which you are interested. Professional organizations, special interest groups, and journals provide not only practice and professional resources, but also contact information for authors and leaders through their websites. These create networking opportunities when their expertise relates to an area of your interest. Your own publications in newsletters and journals may draw contacts, not only with editors and guest editors but also with those who read your work.

Service opportunities abound, not just in your community or through alumni/ae groups at your alma mater, but within public health and international service organizations—volunteers are always welcome. Anytime you have a chance to contribute in ways that are meaningful to you and meet new people, you have ready-made opportunities for networking. These contacts may not all seem career- or work-related to you, but many opportunities for growth and skill development arise from sources you may not have expected.

Electronic mailing lists, commonly called Listservs, are a convenient way to reach out to a large number of people who are interested in a given topic area. One of the many electronic mailing lists you may find of value to you is the CNS Listserv, which can be joined by sending a blank e-mail to cns-listserv-on@ mail-list.com from the e-mail account where you wish to receive messages. An electronic mailing list is a network of people who share questions, answers, examples from their practice, and their thoughts about various topics. Posts from members are received as e-mails to which you can choose to respond if you have something to contribute. You can post your own questions as well, and gain thoughts, support, and sometimes examples of tools or protocols from a wide network of colleagues, sometimes from all over the world. As with most services, protocols for use are shared when you join, and "lurking" for a short while will teach you the usual formats and communication norms of the group (Thede, 2007).

Internet and social media opportunities for networking are increasing exponentially. A thorough discussion is beyond the scope of this chapter, but representative forums are discussed with the note that this is an ever-changing landscape. Chat rooms and bulletin boards may help you make contact with others who share your interests. These websites are often organized around a broad topic focus. Bulletin boards are websites where members post discussion threads and others post comments. Some chat rooms and bulletin boards require you to become a member to access the messages. Others are in the public domain and are accessible to all.

Blogs are longer narrative postings created by an individual. These may relate the individual's experiences or thoughts and opinions around a topic. Bloggers commonly post these monologs on a regular basis, and readers have the opportunity to post their comments and views in response. Blogs may create a networking opportunity if you find bloggers you admire. You can leave comments about their blogs on a regular basis, and they will learn to recognize those who leave thoughtful comments. Bloggers like to help people in their blog community, so if you have a request and they recognize you from your comments, you have made a useful contact.

Twitter is a form of microblogging, limited to 140-character postings. Hashtags are a form of information curation to locate topics and groups. You can follow communities, including the Healthcare Communications and Social Media group (#HCSM) or a nursing site (#RNCHAT), or you can follow nurses who tweet. Twitter events may be scheduled conversations about a specific topic or comments posted ad hoc (Dawson, 2013).

Some social media sites are primarily that: social. A person's network is often family, friends, and other acquaintances and the types of postings are more about social events, life events, and entertainment. Be very aware that what you put out into social media networks reaches far beyond your friend group, and lives on in repostings and comments so that your social media footprint is far larger than you might imagine. A good rule of thumb is to never post anything you'd be embarrassed to post on a public bulletin board. Employers have been known to follow a potential employee's social media, and the impact on hiring decisions can be significant. Health Insurance Portability and Accountability Act (HIPAA) violations and other inappropriate sharing have occurred with negative repercussions on people's academic goals, employment, and license (George, Rovniak, & Kraschnewski, 2013). Many nursing organizations have statements on social media. If you are looking for one, try the National Council of State Boards of Nursing (NCSBN; www.ncsbn.org).

However, social media is also a growing source for continuing professional development, sharing information and thoughts on practice issues and research findings, and networking. Even platforms that began as purely social, such as Facebook, have numerous professional organizations and groups that you can join. You can search on organizations, journals, or topics such as ethics and find forums for learning and networking. Keeping your "social" and "professional" groups and accounts separate is a great way to limit some potentially unwanted exposure.

LinkedIn is a career-focused professional site with a worldwide network. A profile here lists your work skills, and is a way to connect for employment opportunities or with others with similar interests (Zaber, 2013). There are a number of other professional networking sites often focused around a specific profession, theme, or topic of interest. You might notice whether the site you are interested in is sponsored, because a sponsor might sell advertisers access to site members.

A widely used social network is the media-sharing site YouTube, where videos are posted on virtually any topic. Health professionals may find or post educational videos here that you might find helpful in explaining complex content or demonstrating procedures. Other educational web media-sharing sites include podcasts, the Khan Academy, and massive open online courses (MOOCs), each with opportunities to connect with others relating to the content (Grajales, Sheps, Ho, Novak-Lauscher, & Eysenbach, 2014).

As in everything found on the Internet, you'll want to make sure you are relying on credible sources, protecting yourself from privacy invasion, and acting in an ethical way. Always identify yourself on professional sites, be clear whether you are representing your own thoughts or your employer's, and disclose any bias in what you are communicating. Comply with applicable laws and copyrights, knowing that what you post is discoverable (Ventola, 2014).

NETWORKING WITH INDUSTRY

The CNS often has many opportunities to work with representatives from industry. Sales representatives and clinical experts from a variety of pharmaceutical, technological, and medical product companies seek out the CNS either to promote their products or to provide educational support for safe, appropriate use of their products. While this is a valuable resource, do not ignore the additional networking opportunities these contacts provide. There are multiple opportunities here, ranging from influencing product development and participating in pre- or postmarket research, to working as an educational consultant, or even potential employment. These representatives can also be tapped to exhibit at and financially support educational programs or conferences you may be coordinating. If you are seeking contacts in industry, you can contact them through Internet sites or meet them in the exhibit hall at professional conferences.

BENEFITS OF NETWORKING

The benefits of networking will be realized in day-to-day work as a CNS, through skill development, professional opportunities, career mobility, and personal satisfaction. While the relationships you develop within your organization will facilitate your involvement in the right projects and the success of your initiatives, the connections developed outside your workplace will provide an opportunity to compare practices across a wide range of settings. The creative strategies, barriers and how to address them, and outcomes from practice changes accomplished by others can provide depth to your planning and increase your successes. At the very least, you will gain valuable information to enrich your practice and bring new ideas to your workplace (Nicholl & Tracey, 2007).

Collaboration and mentoring opportunities result from networking. You can find opportunities to hone presentation skills or develop competencies in publishing or editorial work. A mentor may help you expand your research skills or provide opportunities for collaborative research. You may find opportunities for funding or learn about fellowships. Communication with leaders and others with diverse perspectives and participation in dialogue about professional trends and national issues will further develop your perspective and the depth of your thinking. Connections can lead to involvement and leadership roles in community activities and professional organizations as well as involvement in legislative or regulatory activities. You can find opportunities to serve as a mentor yourself, sharing your expertise with others.

The relationships you build may result in role expansion with joint appointment as clinical or academic faculty. Employment and entrepreneurial opportunities may come your way. If you are interested in relocating to another city, connections you make can give you a personal insight into that community or hospital as well as local support as you are getting established in your new community.

Once you have established solid relationships, there is even the opportunity to actively engage selected individuals in projects of your own. You might seek individuals from your network to contribute to a journal issue for which you are serving as guest editor, or as speakers at a conference you are working to organize. Rich, Hart, Barrett, Marks, and Ruderman (1995) describe a group of CNSs who formed a peer consultation group. The purpose of the group was to continue to learn together and support one another in professional development. Typical activities included group consultation about clinical situations and group mentoring around professional skill development, such as presentation skills. Ward (2006) describes creating a network focused on developing new approaches to shared problems. He purposefully recruited a cadre of people who would engage in learning activities, discussion, and group projects as a way to challenge themselves to develop new approaches to their work. Ward assigned specific literature, posed questions, and assigned individual and group tasks for the purpose of stimulating thought and creativity within his group. Experimentation was encouraged. The goal was to develop a network of innovative thought leaders. Perhaps one of these examples triggers your own ideas of how you might engage selected members of your network to achieve shared goals.

Networking not only opens doors, it helps you develop so you can confidently step through those doors and contribute in a multitude of ways to the growth of the profession. The resulting experiences will enrich your career in countless ways.

REFERENCES

Dawson, N. (2013, May, June, July). The professional side of social media. *Virginia Nurses Today*, p. 12.

George, D. R., Rovniak, L. S., & Kraschnewski, J. L. (2013). Dangers and opportunities for social media in medicine. *Clinical Obstetrics and Gynecology, 56*(3), 453–462.

Grajales, F. J., Sheps, S., Ho, K., Novak-Lauscher, H., & Eysenbach, G. (2014). Social media: A review and tutorial of applications in medicine and health care. *Journal of Medical Internet Research, 16*(2), e13. doi:10.2196/jmir.2912

Kleinpell, R. M., & Hravnak, M. M. (2005). Strategies for success in the acute care nurse practitioner role. *Critical Care Nursing Clinics of North America, 17*, 177–181.

Nicholl, H., & Tracey, C. (2007). Networking for nurses. *Nursing Management, 13*(9), 26–29.

Rich, B. W., Hart, B., Barrett, A., Marks, G., & Ruderman, S. (1995). Peer consultation: A look at process. *Clinical Nurse Specialist, 9*(3), 181–185.

Scott, D. E. (2007). Networking series part I: Networking fundamentals for nurses. *Wyoming Nurse, 20*(3), 12.

Thede, L. Q. (2007). Networking via e-mail. *CIN: Computers, Informatics, Nursing, 25*(5), 251–253.

Ventola, C. L. (2014). Social media and health care professionals: Benefits, risks, and best practices. *Pharmacy and Therapeutics, 39*(7), 491–499, 520.

Ward, D. (2006). Project Blue Lynx: An innovative approach to mentoring and networking. *Defense AT&L* (July–August), 34–37. Retrieved from http://www.thefreelibrary.com/-a0148756156

Women Into the Network. (n.d.). *What is networking and how can it be of benefit to my business?* Retrieved from http://www.womenintothenetwork.co.uk/page/howtonetwork.cfm

Zaber, M. B. (2013). The benefits of LinkedIn for nursing professionals. *The Maryland Nurse News and Journal, 14*(3), 18.

CHAPTER 19

Facilitating Transitions of Care

PAULA A. O'HEARN ULCH
MARY M. SCHMIDT

If health care settings are islands, the transitions between them are the rolling, foamy waters, waiting to swallow patients up in a sea of uncoordinated care, miscommunication, and service breakdown. Described as vulnerable points of care exchanges with great potential for contributing to unnecessarily high rates of health services use, health care spending, and fragmented care (Naylor, Aiken, Kurtzman, Olds, & Hirschman, 2011), care transitions are a major focus of health care today. Health care systems are trying to create the ideal boat to ferry the patient safely from one level to the next level of care. Many models of care across the transitions have been created, tested, and proven effective in ensuring safe and successful transitions. In each variation of transitional care, the unifying theme is that transitional care includes: (a) movement of patients within the health care environment and community; (b) a comprehensive care plan; (c) time-limited interventions; (d) patient/family participation; and (e) care coordination.

Transitional care interventions focus on patient need, chronic illness management, and reducing risk for readmission and poor outcomes. Transitional care has been implemented in acute care, focusing on the transitions within hospital environments, the goals of which may include maintaining the patient's functional status and improving readiness for discharge. Community-based models of transitional care focus on the hand-offs between hospital to home, subacute/rehabilitation facility, or extended care facility. These models may measure readiness for discharge, as well as outcomes such as patient management of chronic illness, partnering with the community providers, information sharing across settings, and readmission reduction. Each model, regardless of setting, is able to be replicated, in pieces or in its entirety, to be implemented to match the needs of the population, location, and organizational goals for transitional care. In 2012, the National Association of Clinical Nurse Specialists (NACNS) created a taskforce to address the clinical nurse specialist (CNS) role in transitional care. The NACNS website (www.nacns.org) provides information on transitional care, including definitions, descriptions of transitional care, and detailed specifics of several models of transitional care.

ELEMENTS OF TRANSITIONAL CARE

Transitional care cannot succeed without care coordination, which is defined by the American Nurses Association (ANA) as (a) ensuring that patients' needs and preferences are met over time, respective to health services and information sharing across settings, and (b) the purposeful organization of care activities among the patient and involved providers, for appropriate delivery of health care services (Camicia et al., 2013). As a patient moves within the health care setting, coordinated delivery of care and services among providers (focusing on patient need and participation) promotes seamless, cost-effective, and quality care. Nursing, by virtue of education and proximity to the patient, is the role most suited to lead the coordination effort. The Institute of Medicine (IOM) report, *The Future of Nursing: Leading Change and Advancing Health,* stated that "care coordination is one of the traditional strengths of the nursing profession, whether in the community or the acute care setting" (IOM, 2011, p. 94).

As the patient moves within the health care system and community, a team approach, facilitated by the CNS, is fundamental for care coordination and transitional care. The collaborative team, comprising the engaged patient and interdisciplinary providers, is an identified central concept in transitional care.

As the accountable coordinator, the CNS leads the team and facilitates plan development and implementation. The plan, goals, and follow-up recommendations are communicated to all people involved at both the current and future care settings to avoid gaps or duplication of care. Identified and respected as the center of the transitional care effort, the patient and significant others know who is overseeing the plan as the patient moves in and out of the health care system, the extended care setting, or returns home (Snow et al., 2009).

Education of the patient and health care providers is a key component. Patients, family, and providers experience anxiety during care transitions, resulting from a lack of understanding and preparation for self-care, confusion related to conflicting directions, a sense of disregard for their contribution in the care plan, and no identified health care professional to oversee the transition (Snow et al., 2009). CNS involvement and coordination during care transitions present opportunities for patients and providers to learn from one another while developing a better understanding of, and strategies for, a safe transition, thereby reducing anxiety.

Partnerships, built on mutual trust and respect, are essential for team-based transitional care. These partnerships are multidimensional, including the patient, CNS, health care providers, and supportive community personnel. Each partner is aware of his or her role and trusts that the others own their contribution to the safe transition. Given the opportunity to participate, the patient becomes engaged and supportive of the plan and outcome.

As the speed and complexity of health care increase, even the most straightforward of situations may require multiple transitions, between home care services, specialty providers, pharmacies, and durable medical equipment (DME) providers. Therefore, transitional care needs should be assessed in all patients seeking care, regardless of reason or location for meeting with a health care provider. Each interface with the health care system presents an opportunity to assess and support the patient's ability to implement the plan of care, be it surgical recovery, medication changes, management of a new diagnosis, or scheduling follow-up appointments. Each assessment and intervention is targeted at avoiding readmissions and preventing negative outcomes.

The expertise of the CNS lends itself to the care of vulnerable, chronically ill populations at risk for poor outcomes. The CNS role in transitional care focuses on a comprehensive plan of care developed by an interdisciplinary team. The plan is aimed at stabilizing physical health status, and improving the health management and functional ability of complex, vulnerable, chronically ill patients, preventing deterioration and readmission. The centrality of the CNS in transitional care is supported by the NACNS, which adopted the position that the "CNS is educated and prepared to be not only a participant in care coordination but also to partner with other providers in the leadership role for coordination of care transitions" (National Association of Clinical Nurse Specialists [NACNS], 2013).

CNS ROLE IN TRANSITIONS OF CARE

The role of the CNS in transitions of care is described, in the following paragraphs, in terms of plan development, implementation, and systems leadership. Exemplar 19.1 describes the role in its entirety.

Exemplar 19.1

Bob is a 71-year-old gentleman, retired and divorced, with frequent hospitalizations due to exacerbation of severe chronic obstructive pulmonary disease (COPD). Complicating his situation is obstructive sleep apnea (OSA), hypertension (HTN), diabetes mellitus (DM), anxiety, and history of sudden death.

He was originally discharged with a referral to Margaret, a clinical nurse specialist (CNS) providing transitional care in the community. At that time he was considered "noncompliant" with his medications and continuous positive airway pressure (CPAP) usage. He was instructed to follow up with his primary care physician (PCP) and pulmonologist, but had not been given direction related to diabetic management, despite the fact he was taking steroids to manage his respiratory status.

In working with Bob, Margaret extended herself in an authentic and caring way to establish a relationship built upon mutual respect and goals. A plan of care was developed, which was reflective not only of his medical needs, but also of Bob's social and psychosocial needs. Bob's goal was "symptom management." He was tired of feeling short of breath and scared all the time. In order to make this happen,

(continued)

Exemplar 19.1 (continued)

Margaret needed to address his CPAP usage and respiratory treatment plan. Through expert assessment, it became apparent that Bob thought the mask was uncomfortable. As he didn't see the purpose for using the CPAP, the discomfort of the mask outweighed using the machine. Margaret worked with the durable medical equipment (DME) provider to have Bob fitted with a different mask and helped Bob to understand the risks/benefits of CPAP use. When that provider did not respond to her requests, Margaret needed to work with Bob's insurance company to identify an alternate in-network DME provider, and then connected with the new provider, visiting Bob at home to address the issue of the uncomfortable mask and to review CPAP use.

Bob's anxiety and depression played a significant role in the management of his COPD exacerbation. Through regular inquiry, Margaret explored his openness to scheduled anxiolytics and coached him to advocate for that in the PCP office.

As his respiratory status worsened, Bob's functional status gradually diminished and he became increasingly home bound and isolated. To counter that, Margaret facilitated the pulmonologist's recognition of this development and a referral to pulmonary rehabilitation. When the order was entered, pulmonary rehab was scheduled at an inconvenient location. Margaret worked the system to have the location changed and Bob was assessed by the pulmonary rehabilitation nurse.

Bob had a positive relationship with his endocrinologist who was a provider in another health system in the city. Margaret was challenged to cross health systems to facilitate communication of Bob's treatment plan among the PCP, pulmonologist, and endocrinologist in order to establish a collaborative plan of care.

In creating the plan of care with Bob, Margaret discussed end of life planning and treatment wishes. She involved Scott, Bob's son with whom he lives. Bob has three sons, but Scott helps his dad by assisting with medication management and coordinating appointments.

At one point, Bob's anxiety and shortness of breath worsened to the point of needing an acute care admission. At this time, Margaret communicated with Sara, the inpatient CNS, to ensure that the plan of care, initiated in the community, would be woven into the inpatient plan. Sara took the hand-off from Margaret and developed an authentic therapeutic relationship with Bob. Sara and Bob reviewed the community-based plan of care to validate continued accuracy specific to his medications, social supports, concerns, goals for self-management, and community barriers/issues. Sara gathered input from the inpatient providers, and revised the plan, tailoring it to the inpatient setting. Bob had not yet had a chance to be enrolled in pulmonary rehabilitation and was vacillating about his decision and willingness to participate. Recognizing the need for quick intervention to foster engagement (before he changed his mind), Sara brought the pulmonary rehabilitation nurse to his bedside to meet Bob and begin incorporating pulmonary rehabilitation services into the plan of care.

In the past, Bob tested positive for methicillin-resistant *Staphylococcus aureus* (MRSA), which was noted in the medical record along with the need for isolation. This

(continued)

Exemplar 19.1 (continued)

was problematic for Bob. He was concerned that his strength and functional status was deteriorating while he was isolated in his hospital room for a week. It was up to Sara to question that old lab report—validate the existence of MRSA or request an updated test—and to challenge the "isolation rule" that Bob could not leave his room or to challenge the staff (nursing, therapy) to bring a piece of exercise equipment to his bedside to give Bob a chance to stretch his legs, provide a diversion, ease his mind, and maintain his preadmission level of functioning.

Because Bob's eating habits in the community were irregular, his diabetes was managed using short-acting insulin. During the hospitalization, he was taking long-acting and short-acting insulin, which controlled his blood sugars. Bob now needed education to prepare for his discharge home. He needed to know how to resume his insulin regimen and how to plan his meals. To better understand Bob's skill for self-management, Sara inquired about his usual meals, managing his diet and diabetes, and using prednisone. Sara shared this information with the team at daily rounds for planning Bob's transitional care and to ensure a safe hand-off to the next level of care, in the home.

Upon Bob's return home, Sara handed the plan of care off to Margaret, reviewing the updated plan, documenting interventions, outcomes met, and outstanding issues. Margaret, upon her initial home visit postdischarge, reviewed the latest iteration of the plan for accuracy and reflectiveness of Bob's wishes. Recognizing Bob's concern about the increasing length of his hospital stay, Margaret reviewed Bob's understanding of his current health status, verifying his goals for health and self-management skills. Based on this discussion, Bob and Margaret mutually developed outcomes and revised the plan of care. As he was again tapering prednisone, Margaret worked with Bob to manage his blood sugars with the short-acting insulin. Originally, Bob's endocrinology appointment was 6 months from his discharge. Margaret coached Bob on the value of earlier follow-up and facilitated Bob to reschedule the follow-up appointment within 2 weeks after discharge. At this and subsequent provider appointments, Margaret ensured that the plan of care was updated, and that Bob and his physician understood the plan of care.

CNS Role in Plan Development

"A CNS is most likely to care directly for a patient whose diagnosis or care is complex, unique or problematic" (Hamric, Hanson, Tracy, & O'Grady, 2014, p. 370). In becoming involved in the care of patients with a history of discharge failure, whether in the acute care setting or the community, the CNS works to identify the primary reasons for readmission and to alleviate the barriers to success in the community. The expert assessment by the CNS often unearths overlooked details, such as chaotic or unstable housing, knowledge deficits, financial limitations, delivery issues, or repeated failures in transportation, which may explain the patient's behaviors with greater clarity. The assessment may include depression and cognitive screening, health literacy, and quality and reliability of social support, any one of which would impact the patient's ability to engage in and follow the plan of care.

The plan of care begins with the development of the therapeutic partnership between the CNS and the patient. Incorporating a holistic perspective into crafting the plan of care, the CNS acknowledges the patient's personhood and need for self-determination. The CNS mentors staff in how to consider and include the patient as a partner in the team, central to coordinated transitional care. Role-modeling advanced communication skills and respect for an open dialogue ensure patient participation and shared decision making in the development of the plan of care. Basing the plan on individual characteristics, needs, and desires facilitates patient engagement and ensures creation of a plan balanced between best practice standardization and the patient's reality. The ability to personalize his or her own plan of care facilitates the patient's feelings of empowerment and confidence in his or her ability to develop self-management skills necessary for living with chronic illness.

"Collaboration between a CNS and other health care professionals leads to effective and efficient health care" (Hamric et al., 2014, p. 379). Serving as expert consultant, the CNS shares personal experiences and insights into care coordination while collaborating with providers and staff in the acute care, outpatient, and community settings. The medical component of the plan of care is generated by facilitating multidisciplinary collaboration and providing patient-specific consultation to help the health care providers understand the patient's willingness, abilities, and limitations to engage with the prescribed plan. The CNS can gather and integrate the insights of many individuals with differing perspectives into the plan of care. For the acute care CNS, this can occur during daily rounds. In the community, the CNS accompanies the patient to select provider appointments to communicate the existing plan and incorporate the providers' perspectives into plan revision. The plan of care may include mobilizing specialty providers or departments, acute care, or community resources. As a clinical expert, the CNS may intervene by identifying and suggesting creative alternatives to create a successful plan, or by facilitating timely referrals to other members of the multidisciplinary team to achieve outcomes (Hamric et al., 2014). The CNS, with the ability to see the broad perspective and anticipate the disease trajectory, recognizes the need to modify the plan as the patient moves along the trajectory. The elements of the plan must also include the patient's perspective on end-of-life planning.

Success in a plan of care is dependent on outcomes that are realistic and attainable. It may be the CNS's role to act as the voice of reason in stressing realistic outcomes; for example, for a patient with diabetes mellitus (DM) who never monitors blood sugars, setting a goal for complete reversal and four-times-daily monitoring is not realistic. Instead, the CNS could propose a goal of twice daily monitoring initially, gradually building up to the preferred four times daily. Setting goals that are attainable and tailored to the patient will increase the patient's motivation to participate.

The comprehensive plan of care serves as a prescription for the health care team and the patient, and includes information about who is accountable for what aspect of the plan; for example, does the cardiologist or the primary care provider (PCP) manage the warfarin? Is the endocrinologist or the PCP managing the DM? The plan also includes discharge elements including next steps in terms of patient/family education, provision of DME, medication changes, and medical follow-up. The CNS ensures that the accountable individual—patient, pharmacy, provider, and so forth—accepts responsibly and follows through accordingly, and that interventions are necessary and effective in achieving outcomes.

A plan of care is effective only if all participating members know the plan. To that end, the CNS puts much effort and time into communicating and ensuring understanding of the transitional plan. Communication must occur among acute care departments, the acute care setting, and all facets of the community with which the patient will interface—provider clinics, the setting to which the patient is being discharged (if not home), home care, and DME agencies. It is common for the CNS to align with the patient in facilitating communication among providers—a confident, informed patient is able to participate in communicating the plan of care. The communication process is much easier with an electronic health record that ties the settings together. The plan that flows between the acute care setting and the community must be made as visible as possible.

CNS Role in Plan Implementation

The CNS in transitional care provides ongoing surveillance of the patient, monitoring clinical response to treatment, promoting clinical stability, and ensuring early intervention with developing symptoms. Communicating the clinical response to providers is necessary to update and to revise the patient's plan of care. The CNS coaches nursing staff to include evidence-based interventions in the plan of care and make revisions based on an individual patient situation.

The CNS is actively involved in educating and coaching the patient in how to carry out the plan. By understanding the patient's motivation for adhering to the plan, the CNS is able to leverage this knowledge to facilitate behavior change and outcomes achievement. The CNS either provides education or facilitates experts (e.g., certified DM educators or pulmonary rehabilitation nurses) to educate the patient.

The CNS uses the partnership with the patient to increase the patient's confidence and ability in health management, self-advocacy, resource mobilization, and navigation within the health care system. The patient who is confident in heart failure management will contact a provider when there is unanticipated weight gain rather than waiting until additional symptoms develop, resulting in an emergency department visit or avoidable hospitalization. The patient can then incorporate provider instructions into the plan of care (e.g., increase the diuretics for a day or two) and avoid undesirable outcomes (e.g., worsening symptoms and hospitalization).

The holistic assessment, conducted by the CNS, may reveal logistics or system barriers to the plan, such as transportation or parking issues with follow-up appointments, pharmacy prior authorization, or delivery concerns. By identifying the barriers, the CNS is able to work with the patient, provider, and system to reduce or eliminate barriers. Appreciating the challenge a provider has between schedule constraints and time spent with the patient, the CNS coaches the patient in better understanding of the provider's role and consults with the provider to prepare for a focused visit, thereby resolving the time issue and resulting in an efficient and effective patient/provider visit.

The building of relationships and partnerships across settings is instrumental for successful transitional care. The CNS uses advanced skills in forming authentic partnerships and is positioned within the health care system and in the community to foster a team approach and connect the points of transition. The CNS uses leadership skills in building a team based on mutual respect, team learning, and professional accountability, as the CNS facilitates understanding of multiple disciplines' disparate priorities and negotiates alignment of the differing perspectives. "This mediation benefits patients, promotes communication and creates an environment that fosters collaboration" (Hamric et al., 2014, p. 379). Time spent in resource mobilization and community collaboration allows the CNS to assist the patient in identifying supports, informal or formal, that are available to help him or her implement the plan.

The challenge in transitional care is the dynamic nature of the plan of care. Each provider with whom the patient interfaces may revise or update components of the plan. As health conditions change, specific services or necessary follow-up may become less or more frequent; medication regimens are altered. It is essential that all contributors to the plan, including the patient, feel ownership in communicating changes. Equally important is the need for providers to assume responsibility for asking about any recent changes. Written documentation is an effective means to communicate plan changes, allowing the patient to retain and carry this information from provider to provider. When the patient is admitted to the hospital, the plan of care should be reviewed and carried forward from the community, and, upon discharge, the plan is again updated and carried forward from the acute care setting.

CNS Role in Systems Thinking and Leadership

As a leader, the CNS champions opportunities to improve patient care, advance nursing practice, and challenge the health care system to modify current delivery of services. Building on education and clinical expertise, the CNS creates a leadership toolbox, consisting of, for example, diplomatic communication skills, expert consultation, mentorship, role modeling, acting as a change agent, and global awareness. The CNS uses these tools to link disciplines forming collaborative interdisciplinary teams for transitional care.

Transitional care is a critical point in health delivery. With the ability to cross boundaries and see the broad picture, the CNS is positioned to evaluate transitional care, identifying barriers or gaps within the plan or implementation process and challenging the system to solve these issues. The CNS leads the interdisciplinary team in reviewing lessons learned and implementing performance improvement initiatives. Throughout this process, the CNS mentors and empowers team members to own their discipline/specialty's responsibilities for practice changes to address breakdowns in service and transitional care delivery.

An essential component of facilitating transitional care is the communication of the plan among patient, provider(s), and community agency personnel. The electronic health record continues to evolve for enhanced communication across a health care system. The development of a platform to communicate the plan and to coordinate care within the health system and community is instrumental for an efficient transitional care process. As the CNS evaluates transitional care and reviews lessons learned, he or she discovers additional information that, in the role of change agent, is useful for the CNS in collaborating with the interdisciplinary team, informatics specialists, and system leaders to solve issues, close gaps, and create a format to communicate a coordinated and realistic plan of care along the care continuum.

The CNS mentors nursing staff to develop and implement a patient-centered plan for transitional care. The CNS role-models behaviors acknowledging the patient as a whole person, rather than simply identifying the reason for admission. The CNS fosters growth of nursing practice as he or she coaches the staff to develop a therapeutic patient partnership and collaborative approach with caregivers for a coordinated plan incorporating the patient's unique circumstance.

The CNS provides expert consultation to health care and community personnel to bridge the two environments for transitional care. The CNS uses diplomacy when the need for practice change is communicated and team members are challenged to elevate the individual discipline's participation and accountability for transitional care (Table 19.1).

Health care transitions pose a significant challenge for patients, providers, and health systems. Simply moving from one level of care to another places the patient at risk for fragmentation of care and service. The CNS is an expert in clinical practice, collaboration, consultation, coaching, global thinking, and systems leadership. As a health care leader, the CNS should be in the center of a system's effort to address care transitions, leading and partnering in the development and implementation of a transitional plan of care.

TABLE 19.1 Summary of the CNS Role in Facilitating Transitions of Care

Development of the Plan of Care
- Establish therapeutic partnership with the patient
- Explore patient's goals and perceptions of health state
- Collaborate with health care team members to incorporate input into the plan
- Explore end of life goals, as appropriate
- Develop realistic and attainable goals
- Identify and communicate individual accountabilities
- Identify next steps for patient/family—follow-up care, medication management, and so on

(continued)

TABLE 19.1 Summary of the CNS Role in Facilitating Transitions of Care (*continued*)

Communication of the Plan of Care
- Written plan, computerized
- Provide the patient with a copy of the plan
- All health care team members have a copy of the plan
- Attending rounds, office visits, community visits

Implementation of the Plan of Care
- Surveillance of patient: Clinical stability, response to treatment, self-health management
- Communication of patient response, assuring early intervention
- Education and coaching in carrying out the plan of care
- Explore patient's motivation in order to facilitate behavior change
- Role model and coach advocacy behaviors, building patient confidence and skill
- Identify system, logistical, or patient barriers to plan success
- Intervene to reduce barriers
- Mobilize necessary resources to implement plan
- Mentor patient/provider/staff in updating and communicating plan

Systems Thinking and Leadership
- Champion innovative projects or programs
- Change agent—challenge health care system and caregivers to resolve barriers and gaps in care
- Communication skills with diplomacy
- Expert consultation
- Global perspective
- Initiate performance improvement
- Interdisciplinary collaboration—linking disciplines and providers across environments
- Mentor staff to elevate nursing practice, individually and as a whole
- Systems thinking

CNS, clinical nurse specialist.

REFERENCES

Camicia, M., Chamberlain, B., Finnie, R. R., Nalle, M., Lindeke, L. L., Lorenz, L., ... McMenamin, P. (2013). The value of nursing care coordination: A white paper of the American Nurses Association. *Nursing Outlook*, *61*, 490–501.

Hamric, A. B., Hanson, C. M., Tracy, M. F., & O'Grady, E. T. (Eds.). (2014). *Advanced nursing practice: An integrative approach* (5th ed.). St. Louis, MO: Elsevier, Saunders.

Institute of Medicine (IOM). (2011). *The future of nursing: Leading change, advancing health.* Washington, DC: The National Academies Press.

National Association of Clinical Nurse Specialists. (2013). *NACNS position statement on the importance of the clinical nurse specialist role in care coordination.* Retrieved from http://www.nacns.org/html/practice.php#Transitions

Naylor, M. D., Aiken, L. H., Kurtzman, E. T., Olds, D. M., & Hirschman, K. B. (2011). The importance of transitional care in achieving health reform. *Health Affairs, 30*(4), 746–754.

Snow, V., Beck, D., Budnitz, T., Miller, D. C., Potter, J., Wears, R. L., ... Williams, M. V. (2009). Transitions of care consensus policy statement: American College of Physicians–Society of General Internal Medicine–Society of Hospital Medicine–American Geriatrics Society–American College of Emergency Physicians Society of Academic Emergency Medicine. *Journal of General Internal Medicine, 24*(8), 971–976.

CHAPTER 20

Participating in Interprofessional Education

JENNIFER L. EMBREE
JANET S. FULTON

Widespread errors in U.S. health care systems are associated with decreased quality and increased mortality and morbidity. The need to improve health care delivery is well recognized and has been the subject of national efforts to improve both care delivery and education of health care providers (Institute of Medicine [IOM], 2001). One strategy for improving education has been to create mixed or shared educational opportunities for bringing together providers of different professions to achieve common goals. Interprofessional education (IPE) is intended to develop more effective teams and transform health care delivery to safer, more efficient, patient-centered, community-oriented care.

IPE is the purposeful preparation of health professionals for deliberate collaboration by providing students with interactive, interdisciplinary, and structured learning experiences. Until stimulated by legislative initiatives in the Recovery and Reinvestment Act and the Patient Protection and Affordable Care Act, new approaches were limited for achieving better outcomes for chronically ill and at-risk populations. Only small demonstration projects focused on interdisciplinary professional education and team initiatives for managing patients (Kaiser Family Foundation, 2010). These initial efforts at interprofessional collaborative practice in health professions education (HPE) did not succeed in meeting the large-scale need for improvement in practice, and the gap between practice and education continued to widen.

In 2003, the IOM identified five competencies central to health professions education of all future health professions. These IOM competencies are:

- Providing patient-centered care
- Applying quality improvement
- Employing evidence-based practice
- Utilizing informatics
- Working in interdisciplinary teams (IOM, 2003)

With more recent increased emphasis and funding, efforts to strengthen IPE and its sister initiative, Interprofessional Collaborative Practice (IPCP), have been accelerated by increased work around the number of IPE activities in health care schools and IPCP activities in acute care and outpatient care environments.

WHY IPE?

Academic programs preparing health professionals, including nursing schools with all levels of academic programs from prelicensure through doctoral education, are expected to demonstrate some integration of IPE into curricula. IPE is defined as including two or more health or social care students, at a minimum, engaged in learning activities that provide for shared skills, knowledge, understanding, values, and respect for other health care professionals' roles (Barr, Koppel, Reeves, Hammick, & Freeth, 2008; Karim & Ross, 2008). IPE experiences are considered foundational for enhanced cooperation among health care professions (Hammick, Freeth, Koppel, Reeves, & Barr, 2007), and are intended to result in outcome-driven, respectful, positive, collaborative interprofessional team members (Barr et al., 2008; Karim & Ross, 2008).

IMPORTANCE OF IPE DEVELOPMENT FOR IPCP

The desired outcome of IPE is IPCP (Interprofessional Education Collaborative Expert Panel [IECEP], 2011). IPCP is a paradigm shift toward greater integration of care planning within the health care team and away from siloed, profession-specific, and often competing approaches to patient care. Interprofessional practice has unique values, codes of conduct, and ways of working that differ from the historic tradition of profession-centric education (IECEP, 2011). Future IPCP requires continuous interprofessional team competency development for practicing health professionals and students. Interprofessionality is foundational to the core IPCP competency domains and associated specific competencies (D'Amour & Oandasan, 2005; IECEP, 2011). The guiding principles of IECEP are listed in Table 20.1.

WHY IPCP?

IPCP is a partnership between the patient and the health care team. Unlike the "team" of the past that functioned as an unconnected group of providers, an IPCP team has strong partnerships among the team members for shared decision making as well as for collaborative care planning and delivery that includes health and social issues (Canadian Interprofessional Health Collaborative

TABLE 20.1 Guiding Principles and Domains of Interprofessional Collaborative Practice Competencies

IECEP Guiding Principles

Person/people-centered

Civic/people-oriented

Relationship concentration

Process-oriented

Linked with learning activity

Instructive focus

Developmentally appropriate behavioral assessments based on the needs of the learner

Integration across the learning continuum

System context sensitive/applicable across settings

Profession applicability

Language familiar

Professional relevance

Results-focused

From Interprofessional Education Collaborative Expert Panel (IECEP, 2011).

[CIHC], 2010). Conceptually, IPCP hinges on establishing dynamic, goal-driven relationships among professionals in the context of collaboration.

IPCP emphasizes interprofessional provider competencies in four domains: values/ethics for interprofessional practice; roles/responsibilities; interprofessional communication; and teams/teamwork. Corresponding to these domains are broad practice competencies. Each broad competency has a set of more focused competencies. A complete list of the competencies and behavioral expectations can be found in Table 20.2.

Working in the IPCP frame affords an interprofessional team the opportunity for dialogue and pools expertise in achieving collaborative goals for improvement of patient outcomes (IECEP, 2011). Whereas poor interprofessional collaboration negatively impacts the quality of patient care, skills gained through IPE and transferred to IPCP can greatly improve patient outcomes (Zwarenstein, Reeves, & Perrier, 2005).

The complexity of today's health care requires interprofessional team care. Providers working in teams communicate better. Improved communication results in more comprehensive, thoughtful approaches to managing patients' complex and challenging health care needs (IOM, 2001). Although the *accrediting* standards of most professions contain content about interdisciplinary teams, few of these standards include outcomes-based competency expectations. Policy, curriculum, and accreditation changes intended to

**TABLE 20.2 Interprofessional Collaborative Practice
Competency Domains and Competencies**

1. **Values/Ethics for Interprofessional Practice**
   **Work with individuals of other professions to maintain a climate of
   mutual respect and shared values.**
   Behavioral Expectations:
   1. Place the interests of patients and populations at the center of
      interprofessional health care delivery.
   2. Respect the dignity and privacy of patients while maintaining
      confidentiality in the delivery of team-based care.
   3. Embrace the cultural diversity and individual differences that
      characterize patients, populations, and the health care team.
   4. Respect unique cultures, values, roles/responsibilities, and expertise
      of health professions.
   5. Work in cooperation with those who receive care, those who
      provide care, and others who contribute to or support the delivery of
      prevention and health services.
   6. Develop a trusting relationship with patients, families, and other team
      members.
   7. Demonstrate high standards of ethical conduct and quality of care in
      one's contributions to team-based care.
   8. Manage ethical dilemmas specific to interprofessional patient/
      population centered care.
   9. Act with honesty and integrity in relationships with patients, families,
      and team members.
   10. Maintain competence in one's own profession appropriate to scope of
       practice.
2. **Roles and Responsibilities**
   **Use knowledge from one's own role and those of other professions
   to appropriately assess and address the health care needs of the
   patients and populations served.**
   Behavioral Expectations:
   1. Communicate one's roles and responsibilities to patients, families, and
      other professionals.
   2. Recognize one's limitations in skills, knowledge, and abilities.
   3. Engage diverse health care professionals complementary to one's
      own expertise, as well as associated resources, to develop strategies
      to meet specific patient care needs.
   4. Explain roles and responsibilities of other care providers and how the
      team works together to provide care.

(continued)

TABLE 20.2 Interprofessional Collaborative Practice Competency Domains and Competencies (*continued*)

5. Use the full scope of knowledge, skills, and abilities of other health professionals to provide care that is safe, timely, efficient, effective, and equitable.
6. Communicate with team members to clarify each member's responsibility in executing components of a treatment plan or public health intervention.
7. Forge interdependent relationships with professions to improve care/advance learning.
8. Engage in continuous professional and interprofessional development to enhance team performance.
9. Use unique and complementary abilities of all team members to optimize patient care.

3. **Interprofessional Communication**
   Communicate with patients, families, communities, and other health professionals in a responsive and responsible manner that supports a team approach to the maintenance of health and treatment of disease.
   Behavioral Expectations:
   1. Choose effective communication tools and techniques, including information systems and communication technologies, to facilitate discussions and interactions that enhance team function.
   2. Organize and communicate information with patients, families, and health care team members in understandable way; avoid discipline-specific terminology as possible.
   3. Express one's knowledge and opinions to team members involved in patient care with confidence, clarity, and respect, working to ensure common understanding of information, treatment and care decisions.
   4. Listen actively, and encourage ideas and opinions of other team members.
   5. Give timely, sensitive, instructive feedback to others about performance on the team; respond respectfully as a team member to feedback from others.
   6. Use respectful language appropriate for a given difficult situation, crucial conversation, or interprofessional conflict.
   7. Recognize how one's own uniqueness, including experience level, expertise, culture, power, and hierarchy within the health care team, contributes to communication, conflict resolution, and positive interprofessional working relationships.
   8. Communicate consistently the importance of teamwork in patient-centered and community-focused care.

(*continued*)

TABLE 20.2 Interprofessional Collaborative Practice Competency Domains and Competencies (*continued*)

4. **Teams and Teamwork**
   Apply relationship-building values and the principles of team dynamics to perform effectively in different team roles to plan and deliver patient-/population-centered care that is safe, timely, efficient, effective, and equitable.
   Behavioral Expectations
   1. Describe the process of team development and the roles and practices of effective teams.
   2. Develop consensus on ethical principles guiding all aspects of patient care and team work.
   3. Engage other health professionals—appropriate to the specific care situation—in shared patient-centered problem solving.
   4. Integrate the knowledge and experience of other professions— appropriate to the specific care situation—to inform care decisions, while respecting patient and community values and priorities/ preferences for care.
   5. Apply leadership practices that support collaborative practice and team effectiveness.
   6. Engage self and others to constructively manage disagreements about values, roles, goals, and actions arising among health care professionals and with patients/families.
   7. Share accountability with other professions, patients, and communities for outcomes relevant to prevention and health care.
   8. Reflect on individual and team performance for individual, as well as team, performance improvement.
   9. Use process improvement strategies to increase the effectiveness of interprofessional teamwork and team-based care.
   10. Use available evidence to inform effective teamwork and team-based practices.
   11. Perform effectively on teams and in different team roles in a variety of settings.

Adapted from the IECEP (2011).

strengthen teamwork preparation are at various stages of development in the fields of nursing, dentistry, medicine, osteopathy, pharmacy, and public health (American Association of Colleges of Nursing [AACN], 2011). While individual health professions are moving toward incorporating IPCP competency, critical components that the involved professions identify, agree upon, and attempt to strengthen are core IPCP competencies. IPE is becoming embedded into all health professions' educational curricula to guide learning and assessment strategies focused on achieving productive IPE, and ultimately IPCP outcomes (University of Minnesota, 2009).

Health care, with the new emphasis on outcome accountability, especially for chronic disease population management, is requiring providers to shift their lenses to the patient. True patient-centered care occurs when all providers bring the best of their knowledge and skill to advancing health goals for the patient in the context of his or her life and life circumstances. Identifying interprofessional learning approaches to prepare the future health care workforce is critical to making this paradigm shift. Focused workforce retraining that builds interprofessional teams is an effort to improve quality; effectiveness and the safety of care provision are the current challenges (Agency for Healthcare Research and Quality [AHRQ], 2008).

HOW CAN A CNS PARTICIPATE IN IPE?

Where schools are implementing IPE initiatives in the clinical setting, CNSs should be visible as members of the interprofessional team. Students from all the professions should understand the role CNSs have on the team. CNSs should look for opportunities to teach, guide, coach, and mentor students from all the health professions in areas related to their specialty expertise. For example, a CNS with a specialty in wound care might have a medical student shadow for a day. A CNS with a specialty in gerontology could help guide a social work student's assessment of a frail elderly client. Building trust in each other as providers starts with mutual respect grounded in shared experiences. CNSs, with specialty-focused expertise, have much to add to an IPE student experience.

CNSs practice within teams at the patient care, staff, and system levels. CNSs lead interprofessional teams in the design, implementation, and evaluation of evidence-based practice guidelines and standards. Since few practice changes occur without accommodation or engagement of other professions, CNSs are a step ahead in being able to engage in IPE (Zwarenstein et al., 2005). CNSs should involve students in these team initiatives, and use the opportunity to build interprofessional relationships—a secondary goal to developing a new guideline or clinical protocol. These team efforts should also include improved understanding of how interprofessional relationships are central to health care delivery and clinical outcomes.

IPE/IPEC: AN EXEMPLAR

CNSs work across the domains of the patient/client, nursing/nursing practice level, and the organizational/system level—the spheres of influence. The following IPE example about nursing and other providers illustrates the application of the IPE competency domains.

Domain 1: Work with individuals of other professions to maintain a climate of mutual respect and shared values

Once alerted by emergency medical systems (EMS) that a person with a suspected myocardial infarction is en route to the emergency department, an interprofessional code team gets ready, basing their preparedness on the reporting information provided by the EMS staff. The team has learned and practiced in an interdisciplinary learning environment using the principles of IPE. Each member has an assigned role and each member understands his or her individual role and the role of every other member; some roles can be interchanged based on the length and skill set needed during resuscitation efforts. Together the team has a single, focused goal—to deliver competent, coordinated, excellent care that will give the approaching patient the best possible outcome. They learned together, practiced together, debriefed together. Likewise, they have evaluated their collective performance and made improvements in code management. They value and trust each other to provide competent, coordinated care individually and thus collectively.

Domain 2: Use knowledge from one's own role and those of other professions to appropriately assess and address the health care needs of the patients and populations served

The waiting team includes physicians, nurses, a pharmacist, a respiratory therapist, a social worker and a counselor from chaplaincy services. With no hesitation, the patient is moved from the ambulance to the code room and the work continues. Each provider performs effectively and efficiently in a pre-assigned role using language understandable to all professions. Decisions about who does what to accomplish cardiac monitoring, vascular access assessment and potential replacement, respiratory support, need for continued or additional intubation attempts, drug therapy, cardioversion or defibrillation are continually assessed and re-determined. Careful listening and repeating back orders with confidence, clarity, and respect assists in ensuring common understanding of unfolding information and treatment decisions. Team members are results focused and process oriented. Recognizing fatigue in team members, reassignment of roles, and need for additional expertise guide the determination of additional provider inclusion in the resuscitation efforts.

Domain 3: Communicate with patients, families, communities, and other health professionals in a responsive and responsible manner that supports a team approach to the maintenance of health and treatment of disease

During the actual code, team members communicate in an understandable way avoiding discipline-specific terminology and professional jargon that would create confusion or misinterpretation. And while the immediate attention is on the patient, there are team members assigned to find, notify, and support family members with frequent condition updates and questions regarding future care. There are also reports to be completed for the EMS, the paramedics, and admitting services. An efficient code team includes assigned responsibility for these family, system-level, and community components of an unplanned hospital emergency department visit. Assignment of responsibilities takes into account each team member's uniqueness, expertise, culture, power, and hierarchical authority within the team so as to enhance communication, conflict resolution, and interprofessional working relationships.

Domain 4: Apply relationship-building values and the principles of team dynamics to perform effectively in different team roles to plan and deliver patient-/population-centered care that is safe, timely, efficient, effective, and equitable

After the event, the team conducts a debriefing. This process allows everyone on the team to reflect on the whole event and his or her role and role performance. Openly discussing the patient's presentation and treatment, interventions, equipment, and environmental considerations allows the team to build relationships in the spirit of team dynamics and avoids the "blame game." Excellent outcomes are about having the right person for the job in the right place at the right time with the right equipment. If something isn't working well, it's incumbent upon the team to make the changes. No one person should be blamed—it's about shared ownership. Later, a code review team will provide further analysis of the assessments, interventions, and outcomes related to the resuscitation efforts and identify necessary system-level changes based on aggregated code data over time. A CNS typically leads the code review team and provides guidance and facilitates change at the patient, nurse, team, and system levels. The code review team collaborates with those responsible for educational updates and reinforces necessary changes in conjunction with team members.

CNSs should support a care environment that stimulates continuous self-learning, reflective practice, ownership, responsibility, and accountability (National Association of Clinical Nurse Specialists [NACNS], 2004). CNSs are important supports for nursing staff as they engage in IPE/IPEC, helping ensure that they have voice and resources to fully participate. CNSs should role-model constructively, managing conflict about values, roles, goals, and actions among health care professionals and promote accountability for shared health outcomes among interprofessional team members, patients, families, and communities.

HOW TO GET INVOLVED IN IPE

How involved a CNS becomes in IPE will depend on the level of IPE in the clinical setting; however, as IPE expands, it will eventually reach all clinical care settings with student learners. New and experienced CNSs should embrace opportunities to engage in IPE. CNSs can volunteer to work with students in other professions, attend clinical conferences, or serve as a guest discussant or lecturer for topics in their specialty. Sharing the CNSs' expertise is a great way to let others know about the CNS role! Teach through example that the CNS is a specialist in nursing practice for a circumscribed patient population, problem, or diagnosis, but can take that expertise easily to other patient populations as needs arise. Take the time to build a foundation for future health care providers' understanding of the CNS role and practice. Imagine a physician calling a CNS to consult on a complex pain management case or a psychologist seeking support for an innovative outpatient support program. IPE is about building shared values, interpersonal relationships, effective communication, and team practice—real team practice that supersedes listing different providers who have limited understanding of each other's unique contributions.

A CNS can use the competencies of each practice domain (sphere of influence) to become involved in IPE. Begin with a personal needs assessment. Know your personal strengths, clinical expertise, interpersonal style, and emotional intelligence. Be keenly aware of what you do well and lead with your strengths and build relationships. Everyone can improve, but all CNSs have styles and strengths that come more naturally based on personal strengths and emotional intelligence. Focusing on personal strengths and practicing strengths-based leadership tactics also tend to enhance less stellar talents. No one is perfect, so focus on strengths—spend time building strengths. Lead from a position of strength, and surround yourself with others who have different strengths. Interpersonal relationships and collaboration are central to IPE, and ultimately IPCP. Use IPE opportunities to fine tune your skills in relationships and collaboration.

Recognize where problems are occurring in your work setting and consider how IPE and IPCP could assist in problem resolution. Model the way for outcome-driven personal and professional behavior in others. Enlist the support and assistance of other team members and encourage behavior that demonstrates value in other professions. Think team, talk team, and work team. The provider of the future is a team member!

REFERENCES

Agency for Healthcare Research and Quality. AHRQ Health Care Innovations Exchange. (2008, April 14). *Medical team training using crew resource management principles enhances provider communication and stimulates improvements in patient care*. Rockville, MD: Agency for Healthcare Research and Quality. Publication Nos. 08-0034 (1-4). Retrieved from http://www.ahrq.gov/qual/advances2

American Association of Colleges of Nursing. (2011). *The essentials of a master's education in nursing*. Draft. Washington, DC: Author. Retrieved from http://www.aacn.nche.edu/Education/pdf/DraftMastEssentials.pdf

Barr, H., Koppel, I., Reeves, S., Hammick, M., & Freeth, D. S. (2008). *Effective interprofessional education: Argument, assumption and evidence (promoting partnership for health)*. Hoboken, NJ: John Wiley & Sons.

Canadian Interprofessional Health Collaborative. (2010, February). *A national interprofessional competency framework*. Retrieved from http://www.cihc.ca/files/CIHC_IPCompetencies_Feb1210.pdf

D'Amour, D., & Oandasan, I. (2005). Interprofessionality as the field of interprofessional practice and interprofessional education: An emerging concept. *Journal of Interprofessional Care, 19*(S1), 8–20.

Hammick, M., Freeth, D., Koppel, I., Reeves, S., & Barr, H. (2007). A best evidence systematic review of interprofessional education: BEME guide no. 9. *Medical Teacher, 29*(8), 735–751.

Institute of Medicine. (2003). *Health professions education: A bridge to quality*. Washington, DC: The National Academies Press.

Institute of Medicine (US). Committee on Quality of Health Care in America. (2001). *Crossing the quality chasm: A new health system for the 21st century*. Washington, DC: The National Academies Press.

Interprofessional Education Collaborative Expert Panel. (2011). *Core competencies for interprofessional collaborative practice: Report of an expert panel*. Washington, DC: Interprofessional Education Collaborative.

Kaiser Family Foundation. (2010). *Focus on health reform. Summary of new health reform law*. No. Publication #8061. Menlo Park, CA: Author. Retrieved from http://www.kff.org/healthreform/upload/8061.pdf

Karim, R., & Ross, C. (2008). Interprofessional education and chiropractic. *Journal of the Canadian Chiropractic Association, 52*, 766–778.

National Association of Clinical Nurse Specialists. (2004). *Statement on clinical nurse specialist practice and education* (2nd ed.). Harrisburg, PA: Author. Curriculum recommendations on pp. 42–43.

University of Minnesota. Academic Health Center, Office of Education. (2009). *Comparison study of health professional health accreditation standards*. Minneapolis, MN: Author. Retrieved from http://www.interprofessional education.umn.edu/imgs/AccreditationDocFinal030510.pdf

Zwarenstein, M., Reeves, S., & Perrier, L. (2005). Effectiveness of pre-licensure interprofessional education and post-licensure collaborative interventions. *Journal of Interprofessional Care, 19*, 148–165.

PART VI
PROFESSIONAL RECOGNITION

Obtaining Certification: Considering the Options

MELANIE DUFFY

You've come a long way from being an undergraduate in a nursing program to a graduate student in a clinical nurse specialist (CNS) program. You negotiated a job, perhaps wrote your own job description, and figured out where you fit into the organization. Many projects have come your way. New responsibilities and expectations have been placed upon you by others. Now you're probably thinking: What's next? Well, the next step in your professional growth and development is certification. Yes, you've thought about it. You even have colleagues who are certified. But now the time has come for you to take the next logical step in your professional career as an advanced practice nurse (APN).

MEANINGS OF CERTIFICATION

Certification has several meanings depending on the context of the conversation. Certification is not a legal term, however. Professional licensure is a legal term because it is a requirement to practice nursing. Certification, on the other hand, is voluntary. A specific employer may require certification as a condition of employment, but it is not a legal requirement. Certification may have different meanings depending on the state in which you practice. For example, in Pennsylvania certification means that you have been approved by the state board of nursing (SBN) to practice as an APN. Nurse practitioners are certified to practice in the state, but the term connotes approval by the SBN.

Certification carries another meaning. Certification implies protection of the public. The certified CNS has gone above and beyond the basic requirements needed to practice as an APN. The CNS has experience (perhaps years) and advanced knowledge in a specialty area. The CNS has practiced in that specialty and kept abreast of new technologies and treatment modalities. And finally, the CNS has successfully passed a certification examination.

Today's health care consumer is aware of what is involved in the certification process and has added confidence in the certified nurse providing care.

CERTIFICATION AND PROFESSIONAL ORGANIZATIONS

Certification is defined by the American Board of Nursing Specialties (ABNS, 2015) as the formal recognition of specialized knowledge, skills, and experience demonstrated by the achievement of standards identified by a nursing specialty to promote optimal health outcomes. ABNS, a nonprofit membership organization, is focused on improving patient outcomes and protecting the public by promoting specialty nursing certification. ABNS accredits specialty nursing certification examination programs and maintains standards to which certifying nursing organizations adhere. The mission of ABNS is to promote the value of specialty nursing certification. The public recognizes quality nursing care according to the standard of specialty certification (ABNS, 2015).

Many nursing organizations have certification options at different levels. Certification may be available for nurses with specialized practice knowledge and skill, such as in oncology, critical care, or rehabilitation. Nurses are not required to have advanced education at the basic or generalist level of specialty-focused certification. Nurses with associate or bachelor degrees may be eligible for certification. Advanced level certification may be available in the same specialty for nurses with graduate preparation in areas such as oncology CNS or critical care CNS. Some certifying bodies have only one certification option (for the nurse practicing with a basic knowledge of the specialty), while others offer both basic and advanced.

The American Association of Critical-Care Nurses Certification Corporation (AACN cert. corp.) has several certification options available for nurses practicing at both basic and advanced levels. For example, AACN cert. corp. has basic-level certification in the specialty areas of critical care, progressive care, cardiac medicine, and cardiac surgery. AACN cert. corp. has certification examinations available at the advanced level for the CNS providing care to the adult, gerontology, pediatric, and neonatal populations (American Association of Critical-Care Nurses [AACN], 2015a).

The American Nurses Credentialing Center (ANCC), an arm of the American Nurses Association, also has several specialty certifications for the APN. For example, certification is available for CNSs in adult gerontology and pediatrics (ANCC, 2015a). The Oncology Nursing Certification Corporation (2015a) also has an advanced level certification for the CNS—advanced oncology clinical nurse specialist (AOCNS). On a cautionary note, some of the ANCC advanced practice certification exams will be retired after December 31, 2016. The certified nurse will continue to retain certification in the specialty as long as certification criteria are met. However, if the certification lapses, the nurse will not be able to sit for that specific exam in the future. Examples include: adult psychiatric-mental health CNS and child/adolescent psychiatric-mental health CNS (ANCC, 2015a). Other examinations may be affected. Contact the ANCC for clarification.

The National Association of Clinical Nurse Specialists (NACNS, 2005) supports certification at the advanced practice level. The CNS was the first APN to be recognized as having a unique body of knowledge and competencies based on education at the graduate level (Mick & Ackerman, 2002). Verification of advanced knowledge in a specialty area can be accomplished via advanced education at the master's or doctoral level. Most certification options use psychometric examinations to measure knowledge; however, other scientifically sound and legally defensible methods, such as a portfolio, are possible and are being explored for further application (NACNS, 2005). Table 21.1 lists a few examples of currently available CNS certification options.

One problem, as you probably have already surmised, is that there are numerous advanced practice specialties but few certification options for verifying CNS specialty knowledge, but more about that later.

TABLE 21.1 CNS Certification Options

Organization	Title	Credential	Website
American Nurses Credentialing Center	Adult-Gerontology CNS-Board Certified	AGCNS-BC	www.nursecredentialing.org/cert
American Association of Critical-Care Nurses Certification Corporation	Adult-Gerontology CNS (appropriate for Adult-Gero, Pediatric, and Neonatal populations)	ACCNS (ACCNS-AG, ACCNS-P, ACCNS-N)	www.certcorp.org
Oncology Nursing Certification Corporation	Advanced Oncology CNS	AOCNS	www.oncc.org

CNS, clinical nurse specialist.

RATIONALE FOR CERTIFICATION

Why should you become certified? After all, becoming certified means you'd likely have to take a *test* and *pass* it! Well, there is a little bit more to it than just studying for and passing an exam. Consider these data: The Oncology Nursing Society stated that 88% of nurses agreed that certification enhances confidence in clinical abilities and 97% stated certification provides personal satisfaction (Oncology Nursing Society, 2015b). Now talk to your colleagues and ask why they pursued certification. Several reasons in support of certification will be evident. First, certification is validation of your knowledge by a professional body. Yes, you will probably have to study to be successful with the test, but your advanced knowledge is already there. You just have to brush up on a few things.

Second, professional certification demonstrates to the public that the holder of a certification credential has demonstrated knowledge of practice standards in a specialty area. The patient and family recognize that the nurse providing care has the requisite experience, knowledge, and skills to provide care to the complex patient. Boards of nursing often use professional certification as a proxy for knowledge in a specialty and issue a state certificate to practice as an APN/CNS based on professional certification. Certification, such as Adult-Gerontology Clinical Nurse Specialist-Board Certified (AGCNS-BC), is a professional credential. Protection of the public is the state's issue specifically. A state may ask for and/or accept the professional credential as part of a procedure to protect the public. Advanced level certification signals competence, advanced abilities, and confidence to the consumer.

Third, your employer benefits from your certification. A CNS who obtains professional certification contributes to the overall reputation of the health care setting in which he or she practices. Certification and the continuing education required to maintain the credential contribute to an environment of professionalism and retention. The consumer recognizes that the health care setting invests in an APN who has greater accountability for actions and ensures delivery of evidence-based quality care. Liability rates for the employee/employer may decrease (AACN, 2015b).

Fourth, you will have a reputation as a certified CNS. Certification builds self-confidence about knowledge and expertise, and gives you the satisfaction of having achieved a prestigious personal goal. Specialty certification demonstrates a nurse's commitment to career development and dedication to provide optimal care to the patient. Your accomplishment will serve to inspire colleagues to also seek certification. Perhaps you will be the one giving advice to others who wish to pursue certification. Last, some employers provide financial support for certification or incentives to achieve and maintain certification. Check to see if your employer offers financial support for a review course and/or reimbursement for costs incurred to take the exam. Ask about a financial bonus/salary adjustment for successful completion of the exam or if certification will be positively reflected in your annual performance review and/or merit-based salary increase.

THE DECISION IS MADE: TEST-TAKING SKILLS

You finally made the decision to take the plunge! You invested in a review book with sample questions in your specialty. You reviewed the test blueprint, available on most nursing organization websites. Perhaps you became part of a study group so you wouldn't have to embark on the project alone. Maybe you made flash cards with bits and pieces of information that were difficult for you to grasp. Audiotapes were also a good investment since you have a long commute to work and sit in traffic.

How will you actually prepare for the test? Several test-taking strategy books, articles, and web-based resources are available. ANCC has an online course that addresses ways to prepare for the exam, skills to improve the ability to be successful on an exam, and practice questions with answers/rationale (ANCC, 2015b). Dennison and Rollant offer some helpful hints on how to prepare to take the test and be successful (Dennison & Rollant, 2002).

First, use practice questions. Ask why you missed the question if you chose the incorrect answer. Read the question thoroughly. Highlight key points as you read the question. Answer the question after you read the stem without looking at the options. Read all options as well as the stem. Eliminate clearly incorrect options. Eliminate similar options that say the same thing. Choose the answer that matches the question in scope. If the question is general, give a general answer; if the question is specific, give a specific answer.

Second, do not assume information that is not given. All important information is included in the stem. Included information is probably important.

Third, answer the easy questions first. Return to the difficult questions later. Do not leave any questions blank.

Select an answer according to clinical priority. Start with the most life-threatening problems. Think airway, breathing, and circulation. Next consider the seriousness of a complication if interventions are missed. Think long-term consequences and disability. Next, consider pain and comfort. Acute pain is a priority unless a life-threatening situation is present. Actual problems always take precedence over potential problems. Use the nursing process to determine next steps if the question asks what to do next in a situation. Use Maslow's hierarchy of needs to determine the initial need if the question asks what a patient needs. Focus on patient safety if the patient doesn't have an urgent physiologic need. Choose actions to check the patient first and the equipment second. Look at the big picture and the organ systems affected. The pulmonary and cardiovascular systems are the priority in life-threatening situations.

Avoid outright guessing. If you are not sure, first try to eliminate any choices that are obviously or most likely incorrect. Make your best choice from the remaining options.

Maintaining concentration is also a test-taking skill. Rephrase a question rather than rereading the same question over and over. Write down normal lab values or formulas on scrap paper before you answer the first question. Read the answers in reverse order—option *d* to option *a*. Take some slow, deep breaths to refocus and regroup. Or you may find a quick trip to the restroom will facilitate renewed thinking capabilities.

Changing answers—should you or shouldn't you? Be aware of your specific pattern of errors. If you miss questions because you don't read them thoroughly, then of course change the answers. But if you miss questions even though you read them thoroughly, don't change the initial answers.

Budget your time. Generally certification exams provide sufficient time to complete the task. Proceed quickly and carefully through the questions, but don't spend too much time on any one question. You can always come back to it.

Lastly, don't cram the night before the exam. Go to bed at a reasonable time. Wear comfortable, layered clothes the day of the exam. Eat a light, healthy meal—avoid the Danish or donut. Eat something with protein and a little fat to carry you through to the end of the task—perhaps an egg sandwich or an apple with a little peanut butter. And think positively!

NO CERTIFICATION AVAILABLE? NOW WHAT?

Numerous advanced practice specialties exist, but few certification options are available. Why doesn't every specialty have a certification option? Well, for one reason, it is cost prohibitive. To produce a psychometrically sound and legally defensible examination to validate knowledge costs hundreds of thousands of dollars. Most nursing organizations are relatively small, have few members, and can't afford the financial commitment. Grants and donations may be options for examination development but may not be able to support continued maintenance. Examinations are constructed using expert panels that determine the content and write the individual test items. This process is required for initial test development and ongoing test updates. Overall, the ongoing process is very expensive. The expense of developing and offering the certification exam will not be recoverable for small specialty practice groups for which the test takers pool is limited.

So what's the alternative? One option is to successfully complete specialty certification at the basic knowledge level if an advanced version is not available. You still will have demonstrated expertise in a specialty, will be a role model for your colleagues and staff nurses, will have contributed to your institution's reputation, and will have gained financially.

A second option is to demonstrate your knowledge and expertise through submission of a portfolio. A portfolio is a compendium document that reflects practice competencies and may include examples of specific patient cases; projects developed, implemented, and completed; products, equipment, actions of medications, and treatment modalities evaluated; research and evidence-based projects completed; continuing education activities; podium/poster presentations at local, regional, national, and international conferences and professional meetings; and nurses mentored. Collectively, the examples in the portfolio provide a comprehensive and in-depth reflection of an individual's CNS practice.

SUMMARY

Certification is the next logical step in your professional career as a CNS. Do it now. Don't put it off. There's no time like the present. Join your certified colleagues as one with a validated knowledge base and demonstrated expertise in a specialty. Become accountable and responsible for your actions above a basic level. The certification designation will only add to your exemplary career as a CNS.

REFERENCES

American Association of Critical-Care Nurses. (2015a). *AACN certification corporation fact sheet*. Retrieved from http://www.aacn.org/wd/certifications

American Association of Critical-Care Nurses. (2015b). *Nurse certification benefits patients, employers and nurses*. Retrieved from http://www.aacn.org/wd/certifications

American Board of Nursing Specialties. (2015). *ABNS vision, mission, values*. Retrieved from http://www.nursingcertification.org

American Nurses Credentialing Center. (2015a). Retrieved http://www.nursecredentialing.org

American Nurses Credentialing Center. (2015b). Retrieved from http://ancc.learner community.com/products

Dennison, R., & Rollant, P. (2002). *Test-taking techniques: Review and resource manual*. Washington, DC: American Nurses Association, Institute for Research, Education, and Consultation at the American Nurses Credentialing Center.

Mick, D. J., & Ackerman, M. H. (2002). Deconstructing the myth of the advanced practice blended role: Support for role divergence. *Heart and Lung, 31*(6), 393–398.

National Association of Clinical Nurse Specialists (NACNS). (2005). *White paper on certification of clinical nurse specialists*. Retrieved from http://www.nacns.org

Oncology Nursing Society. (2015a). Retrieved from http://www.ons.org

Oncology Nursing Society. (2015b). Retrieved from http://www.ons.org

CHAPTER 22

Navigating the Privileging and Credentialing Process

SUSAN SENDELBACH

Credentialing and privileging are mandated by accrediting agencies; for example, The Joint Commission (TJC), the Accreditation Association for the Ambulatory Healthcare (AAAHC), the National Committee for Quality Assurance (NCQA), and managed care organizations (MCOs), to protect patients ensuring that professionals within the institution are competent and practicing within their scopes of practice (Hravnak, 2009; Kamajian, Mitchell, & Fruth, 1999; Magdic, Hravnak, & McCartney, 2005). It is required whether the CNS is employed by a private group or practice plan or by the hospital itself (Hravnak, 2009). Historically, only physicians were credentialed and privileged. However, in 1983 TJC established new regulations that allowed nonphysician providers on medical staff to practice as allied health professionals (Stanley, 2011). This change allowed the credentialing and privileging of advanced practice registered nurses (APRNs), including clinical nurse specialists (CNSs). The credentialing and privileging process is important to CNSs as it demonstrates our unique education, competence, and value to patient care to physicians and nonclinicians in health care settings (Jones-Schenk, 1998). Each hospital has the responsibility of ensuring that APRNs who practice within their institution are credentialed, privileged, and re-privileged through the medical staff process or a procedure that is equivalent (The Joint Commission, 2015). Although credentialing and privileging are two different processes, they are usually done in parallel.

WHAT IS CREDENTIALING?

The American Nurses Association (ANA) defines credentialing as "the process of assessing and validating the qualifications of a licensed independent practitioner to provide patient care services based on an evaluation of the individual's licensure, training, experience, current competence, and the ability to perform the requested privileges" (American Nurses Association [ANA], 2006). This process is used by health care organizations; it involves obtaining three critical parameters: (1) verification of a CNS's licensure; (2) education and relevant training; and (3) experience, ability, and current competence to perform the requested privileges (The Joint Commission, 2015). Verification of education and relevant training should be obtained from primary sources including, for example, letters from schools documenting satisfactory completion of program requirements or degree conferred (The Joint Commission, 2015). The credentialing process can be conducted by the hospital, through the human resource department or department of medical affairs, or delegated to a credential verification organization (CVO) as specified in the medical staff bylaws of the institution, based on the recommendations of the medical staff, and as approved by the governing body (Kamajian et al., 1999; The Joint Commission, 2015). The overall goal of verifying credentials is to ensure that the applicant's qualifications are consistent with the position's responsibilities and that the applicant is appropriately prepared to perform the duties implied by the credential and to minimize the possibility of granting privileges based on the review of fraudulent documents (Hamric, Hanson, Tracy, & O'Grady, 2013; The Joint Commission, 2015).

WHAT IS PRIVILEGING?

Privileging is the "authorization granted by the governing body of a healthcare facility, agency, or organization to provide specific patient care service within well-defined limits, based on qualifications reviewed in the credentials process" (ANA, 2006). The process includes developing and approving a procedure list; processing the application; evaluating applicant-specific information; submitting recommendations to the governing body for applicant-specific delineated privileges; notifying the applicant and relevant personnel of the privileging decision; and monitoring the use of privileges and quality-of-care issues (The Joint Commission, 2015). The privileges that a CNS requests will differ by state, since all CNSs practice within the scope of practice as defined in the individual state's nurse practice act. The state in which the CNS practices determines the limits and privileges of the CNS license (Fulton, Lyon, Lyon, Goudreau, & Goudreau, 2014; Kamajian et al., 1999). For example, a CNS may or may not need to have a collaborative agreement with a physician to be able to prescribe medications. This would be defined by the state's scope of practice.

The Joint Commission (2015) mandates that the applicant's ability to perform requested privileges be evaluated. This includes documentation that the applicant has no health problems that could affect his or her practice; JC recommends this be confirmed (The Joint Commission, 2015). In addition, when applying for privileges, the National Practitioner Data Bank (NPDB) is queried to potentially discover proceedings and reports against an applicant. The NPDB was created by Congress as a quality and safety measure and contains reports related to malpractice payments and certain actions of health care practitioners, including CNSs (U.S. Department of Health and Human Services, 2014).

As a part of the privileging process, peer recommendation is required and includes written information about the applicant's clinical knowledge; technical and clinical skills; clinical judgment; interpersonal skills; communication skills; and professionalism (The Joint Commission, 2015). An evaluation of the requested information is conducted before recommending approval of privileges. The hospital must have a process to determine if there is sufficient clinical performance to make a decision to grant, limit, or deny the privilege requested by the applicant. A period of focused professional practice evaluation is required for all initially requested privileges, is defined by the organized medical staff, and can include activities such as chart review and monitoring clinical practice patterns. The Joint Commission (2015) also requires that the reprivileging process take place at least every 2 years.

Special considerations of the credentialing and privileging process include an expedited process that may be used for an initial appointment; temporary privileges that allow for temporary clinical privileges for a limited time period; disaster privileges that will allow privileges to volunteers eligible to be licensed independent practitioners; and a process for the practice of telemedicine (The Joint Commission, 2015).

THE CREDENTIALING AND PRIVILEGING PROCESS

The ANA recommends the nursing peer review within the credentialing and privileging process be conducted by other APRNs and suggests one of two models (ANA, 2006). The first is the Nursing Model, in which the nursing peer review committee reviews and makes a recommendation to the chief nursing officer (CNO), who then reviews and credentials the APRN. The second is the Collaborative Model, in which the nursing peer review committee initially reviews and approves the APRN credentialing application consistent with the institution's policy, and final approval is granted by the institution's Credentialing Committee. Regardless of the model chosen, it is important that APRNs be a part of the process in order to support the principle of self-regulation. ANA (2006) views the credentialing and privileging of APRNs, including CNSs, as critical processes that help support the full scope of practice for the APRN. In addition, the Magnet® Standards support the autonomous practice of nurses, including APRNs. As a part of Magnet designation, the American Nurses Credentialing Center (ANCC) asks for a description of the process for "credentialing, privileging, and evaluating advanced practice registered nurses (APRNs), including reprivileging" (2013, p. 28). The CNO must also submit documentation of his or her participation (or designee) in the privileging process for advanced practice nurses (ANCC, 2013). Clearly the credentialing and privileging of APRNs is becoming the standard, as opposed to the exception.

SUMMARY

Although the credentialing and privileging process may seem to be arduous, it is vital to ensure patient quality of care. Additionally, the process promotes the full scope of practice for APRNs and provides for self-regulation of CNSs and CNS practice.

REFERENCES

American Nurses Association. (2006, October 11). *Credentialing and privileging of advanced practice registered nurses.* Retrieved from http://www.nursingworld.org/MainMenuCategories/HealthcareandPolicyIssues/ANAPositionStatements/practice.aspx

American Nurses Credentialing Center. (2013). *2014 magnet application manual.* Silver Springs, MD: American Nurses Credentialing Center.

Fulton, J. S., Lyon, B. L., Lyon, B., Goudreau, K. A., & Goudreau, K. (2014). *Foundations of clinical nurse specialist practice.* New York, NY: Springer Publishing Company.

Hamric, A. B., Hanson, C. M., Tracy, M. F., & O'Grady, E. T. (2013). *Advanced practice nursing: An integrative approach.* St. Louis. MO: Elsevier Health Sciences.

Hravnak, M. (2009). Credentialing and privileging for advanced practice nurses. *AACN Advanced Critical Care, 20*(1), 12–14. doi:10.1097/NCI.0b013e31819435bb

Jones-Schenk, J. (1998). The brave new world of advanced practice: Credentialing and privileging. *Applied Nursing Research, 11*(3), 99–100.

Kamajian, M. F., Mitchell, S. A., & Fruth, R. A. (1999). Credentialing and privileging of advanced practice nurses. *AACN Clinical Issues: Advanced Practice in Acute & Critical Care, 10*(3), 316–336.

Magdic, K. S., Hravnak, M., & McCartney, S. (2005). Credentialing for nurse practitioners: An update. *AACN Clinical Issues, 16*(1), 16–22. doi:00044067-200501000-00003 [pii]

Stanley, J. M. (2011). *Advanced practice nursing: Emphasizing common roles.* Philadelphia, PA: F.A. Davis.

The Joint Commission. (2015). *The Joint Commission comprehensive accreditation and certification manual.* Oakbridge, IL: The Joint Commission.

U.S. Department of Health and Human Services. (2014, October). *Data bank 101 for nurses: A guide to the data bank and how it affects you.* Retrieved from http://www.npdb.hrsa.gov/resources/factsheets/nurses.pdf

CHAPTER 23

Qualifying for Reimbursement

SUSAN DRESSER

National mandates to improve our health care system, growing physician shortages, and changes in reimbursement regulations have all opened new opportunities for clinical nurse specialists (CNSs). CNSs are continually challenged to demonstrate their value by communicating their impact on clinical outcomes, cost savings, and quality improvement. Generating revenue by billing for professional services provided is a relatively new and challenging opportunity for CNSs to demonstrate monetary value. This is a challenge for which most CNSs initially feel unprepared. Findings from a recent study of the National Association of Clinical Nurse Specialists (NACNS) by Zuzelo, Fallon, Lang, and Mount (2004) revealed that while CNSs were generally aware of Medicare structures and processes, many had basic knowledge deficits. Additionally, many lacked an understanding of federal regulations recognizing CNSs as advanced practice registered nurses (APRNs) who could become Medicare providers and bill for services. Their findings suggested that some CNS graduate programs need to incorporate content pertaining to reimbursement methodologies. Navigating the complex, confusing, and always-changing system of rules and regulations inherent in the reimbursement arena can be overwhelming and frustrating, even for the experienced CNS. This chapter provides an introductory overview of the coding and reimbursement processes and some insights from my own personal experience as one of the first CNSs in my state to achieve Medicare provider privileges. A brief history of the legislation that legitimized our current practice is included.

BACKGROUND OF REIMBURSEMENT LEGISLATION

The Omnibus Budget Reconciliation Act of 1989 first gave APRNs the opportunity for reimbursement, although it was restricted to those practicing in skilled nursing facilities and areas designated as rural (Richmond, Thompson, & Sullivan-Marx, 2000). Several years later, President Bill Clinton signed into law the historic Balanced Budget Act (BBA) of 1997. This landmark

215

legislation signified an historic victory for APRNs by increasing and expanding our direct reimbursement opportunities in all settings. With the passage of this law, CNSs were able for the first time in history to be reimbursed by Medicare directly, regardless of geographic location or practice site.

The passage of this law provided new financial opportunities for CNSs to be recognized as key health care providers, and as such, the Act requires that they develop a basic understanding of reimbursement rules and regulations.

THIRD-PARTY REIMBURSEMENT ENTITIES

Depending upon your employment practice agreement, some portion of your revenue as an APRN provider may come directly from health care insurers, known collectively as third-party payers. There are several types of third-party reimbursement entities with which CNSs should be familiar. These include government insurers such as Medicare and Medicaid, commercial insurers such as Aetna, and private health insurance companies such as BlueCross BlueShield. Each of these groups of payers has its own set of rules and criteria defining reimbursement policies, credentialing, contracting, and fee schedules. Understanding the basic reimbursement rules and methods of Medicare is a good starting point because most other third-party payers adopt their rules.

MEDICARE

Medicare was established by Congress as part of the Social Security Act of 1965 primarily to provide a health insurance program for the elderly and disabled. It is administered by the Centers for Medicare and Medicaid Services (CMS) of the U.S. Department of Health and Human Services. Local Medicare carrier agencies administer the four major Medicare programs. Part A, or hospital insurance, covers inpatient hospital services and some skilled nursing home care. Part B covers the services of physicians and other selected providers like CNSs and NPs. Medicare's third program, Part C, is known as Medicare Advantage. This program is made up of managed care plans, preferred provider organizations, and specialty plans and is provided as an alternative coverage to Parts A and B. The fourth program, Part D, covers prescription drug costs (Baker & Baker, 2014).

MEDICAID

Medicaid is the jointly funded and operated federal and state health care program intended to provide health care coverage to low-income individuals and families, the elderly, and the disabled (Baker & Baker, 2014). Each state establishes its own Medicaid rules under broad federal guidelines. Medicaid covers services provided by CNSs in many states.

QUALIFICATIONS, COVERAGE REQUIREMENTS, BILLING, AND PAYMENT FOR MEDICARE SERVICES

If you intend to bill for services provided to Medicare beneficiaries you must first be enrolled as a Medicare provider. Enrollment is the process used by Medicare to grant Medicare billing privileges. To be recognized as a Medicare provider you must meet all of the following requirements:

- Be a graduate of a CNS master's, postmaster's, or doctor of nursing practice (DNP) program of study
- Be a registered nurse currently licensed to practice in the state where you practice and authorized to furnish the services of a CNS according to your state's law
- Be certified as a CNS by an approved national certifying body that has established standards for CNSs (Centers for Medicare and Medicaid Services [CMS], 2015)

The following coverage criteria apply to determine if CNS services are eligible for reimbursement:

- You must be legally authorized and qualified to furnish the services in the state where the service is performed
- Services must be reasonable and necessary and not otherwise precluded due to a statutory exclusion
- Services are typically considered physician's services if furnished by a medical doctor or a doctor of osteopathy
- Services are performed in collaboration with a physician as required by state law
- Surgical assistant services provided by a CNS may be covered
- Incident to services and supplies may be covered (CMS, 2014a, 2014b, 2015)

The types of services a CNS may provide and receive payment are governed by state law and regulations overseeing the CNS's scope of practice in the state in which the service is performed. Examples of services include performing a history and physical examination, interpreting x-rays, or minor surgical procedures.

Medicare reimburses APRNs based on an annually adjusted fee schedule established for physicians, where the amount of payment is predetermined for each service provided. The Medicare Physician Fee Schedule (PFS) is based on a fee-for-service reimbursement structure and was designed to reflect the relative time and intensity of effort associated with providing the various physician services along with practice expenses (Chapman, Wides, & Spetz, 2010). Payment for services provided by a CNS is made at 85% of the amount a physician would be paid under the PFS. Payment for services provided using the incident to provision in a setting outside of a hospital is made at 100% of the PFS. Incident to billing is prohibited if there is no physician on site, for inpatient hospital services, services provided to a new patient, or to a new problem on an existing patient (Brassard, 2015). In an incident-to situation, the physician must perform the initial exam and establish the plan of care for a specific condition/complaint in order for the CNS to then follow up and treat that condition (Dowling, 2014) (Table 23.1). One thing to keep in mind when billing incident-to is that this process masks the services provided by the CNS because the billing is through the physician's national provider identification (NPI) (Chapman et al., 2010).

HOW TO ENROLL IN MEDICARE

CNSs may enroll through the Internet-based provider enrollment, chain, and ownership system (PECOS) or by completing the paper enrollment application (Form CMS-855I). This form and instructions for completing it can be downloaded from www.cms.hhs.gov/MedicareProviderSupEnroll. The CMS-855I form is for APRNs and physicians who provide Medicare Part B services to beneficiaries. Medicare assigns unique provider identification numbers to each of its enrolled health care providers. These NPI numbers are used to identify providers in all Medicare transactions. The enrollment application is used to collect the required documentation to ensure you are qualified and eligible to enroll as a provider and includes professional licenses, the NPI notification letter, evidence of national certification, and evidence of a collaborative practice agreement with a physician. The definition of collaboration defers somewhat to state law in terms of how the exact collaborative arrangement is made. If you are practicing in a state that does not require a collaborative practice agreement, you need only to provide details about how you would communicate with a physician when an issue outside your scope of practice arises. The enrollment process can take up to approximately 60 days, sometimes longer. You may bill Medicare directly using your NPI number or you may have your employer bill for your services using your NPI number. If you bill under the incident-to provision, your supervising physician must bill under his or her NPI number for the service you provide.

CODING FOR PROPER REIMBURSEMENT

Within your practice setting there should be resources available for training on documentation and coding. For those who wish to pursue education on their own, the CMS website is probably the most conclusive and accessible source of information and offers a variety of web-based training courses, educational products, and provider updates in addition to current statutes and regulations. When submitting a bill for service to third-party payers, it is essential to

TABLE 23.1 Common Terms

Term	Stands For	Definition
Collaboration		The process where CNSs work with one or more physicians to provide health care services within the scope of the CNS's professional expertise with medical direction and appropriate supervision as required by the law of the state in which the services are provided. The collaborating physician is not required to be physically present when the services are provided (CMS, 2015).
ICD-9	International Classification of Diseases, 9th edition	A system designed to standardize health care diagnoses for reimbursement purposes
ICD-10	International Classification of Diseases, 10th edition	The current international version of ICD that is used to report diagnoses in all health care settings
CPT Code	Current Procedural Terminology Code	A system designed by the American Medical Association to report diagnostic and surgical services and procedures
RBRVS	Resource-Based-Relative-Value Scale	A discounted fee schedule for Medicare used to reimburse physicians. A payment method that classifies health services in terms of effort, practice expenses, and malpractice insurance
RVU	Relative-Value Unit	A unit of health care that is specifically reimbursed according to rates set by CMS and vary according to level of care and geographical area

(*continued*)

TABLE 23.1 Common Terms (*continued*)

Term	Stands For	Definition
DRGs	Diagnostic Related Groupings	A system of classification for inpatient hospital services based on diagnosis, age, sex, and presence of complications. It is used to identify costs of providing services and as a mechanism for predetermined reimbursement to a hospital based on the patient diagnosis
CMS	Centers for Medicare and Medicaid Services	Federal agency that determines rules and regulations for health care reimbursement policy
FFS	Fee for Service	The traditional health care payment method where providers receive payment for services provided
Fee Schedule		A predetermined list of fees that a third-party payer allows for payment for all health care services
Incident-to Provision		Services performed by a CNS and billed as incident to a physician's service must meet the following requirements: The service must be an integral although incidental part of the physician's service and must be performed under the direct supervision of a physician (in the office suite where the physician is immediately available to provide assistance and direction); the physician must perform the initial, face-to-face, personal service to establish the plan of care; there must be subsequent follow-up services by the physician that reflect active participation in the treatment plan
PPS	Prospective Payment System	A capitated reimbursement plan that provides payment based on designated amount per enrollee per year

CNS, clinical nurse specialist.

understand and comply with documentation requirements. If documentation is incomplete, the payer may refuse payment, which will result in decreased reimbursement revenue. Inadequately documented medical records can also expose the CNS to false-claim liability actions such as Medicare audits, fines, and even criminal prosecution for fraud (Craig, 2014). You can obtain higher levels of reimbursement and minimize the threat of being audited by thoroughly and accurately documenting the care provided to your patients. All payment decisions are made based upon the appropriate documentation and selection of Current Procedural Terminology (CPT), International Classification of Diseases, 10th edition (ICD-10), and evaluation and management (E/M) codes provided. While the details of coding can feel overwhelming, CNSs can and should learn the fundamentals and will benefit greatly by doing so.

CPT CODES

CPT codes are five-digit numeric codes developed by the American Medical Association to describe medical and diagnostic services, procedures, and treatments (Baradell & Hanrahan, 2000). The intent of these codes was to create a standard language to describe and communicate medical, surgical, and diagnostic procedures. CPT codes attempt to provide a consistent, uniform language nationwide for communication among physicians and other health care providers, patients, and third-party payers. To illustrate, there are 10 codes for physician office visits. Five of these codes apply to new patients (99201–99205), and the other five apply to established patients (99211–99215) (Table 23.2).

E/M CODES

The differences between the five codes in each CPT category reflect the level of E/M of a patient. These E/M levels or codes are based on the level of complexity of the visit as indicated by three key components: (a) extent of review of patient history, (b) extent of physical examination, and (c) complexity of medical decision making (Bendix, 2013; Gapenski, 2012). The history includes history of present illness; review of systems; and past, family, and social history. Levels of complexity range from "problem-focused," "expanded problem-focused," "detailed," and "comprehensive. The exam section contains the same four levels of complexity. The medical decision-making element includes "straightforward" or low, medium, or high complexity (Table 23.2). The more detailed or complex the visit, the higher the level of E/M code chosen and the higher the reimbursement. Documentation must support the level chosen and must meet the requirements for that level. Learning the required elements that must be performed in the history and physical exam and reflected in the decision making is one of the more difficult and lengthy processes to master.

TABLE 23.2 Coding for Outpatient Visits: Returning Patient

Elements That Make an E/M Visit	CPT Code 99212	CPT Code 99213	CPT Code 99214	CPT Code 99215
History:	1	1	4	4
History of Present Illness	Problem focused	Expanded problem focused	Detailed	Comprehensive
Review of Systems		1	2	10
Personal, Family, and Social History			2	2
Examination	1	2	5	8
	Problem focused	Expanded problem focused	Detailed	Comprehensive
Medical Decision Making	Straightforward	Low complexity	Moderate complexity	High Complexity
Time Spent	10	15	25	40

CPT, Current Procedural Terminology; E/M, evaluation and management.
Numbers beneath each CPT code indicate the minimum level of complexity (number of required elements) required to bill for each code. Adapted from Bendix (2013).

DIAGNOSIS CODES

International Classification of Diseases codes are used to specify patient diagnoses, which helps to provide the justification or medical necessity for a procedure or service provided. Published by the World Health Organization, ICD codes are used to communicate information about diseases, conditions, symptoms, and injuries with the original intent being to track mortality and epidemics. The ICD-10 code set contains literally thousands of codes that reflect current medical practice and technology. These codes can be from three to seven characters, where the first three indicate a disease category followed by characters that indicate etiology, anatomic site, and severity (Gray, 2014).

HOSPITAL-EMPLOYED CNSs

If you are a CNS employed by a hospital, one of the details you will have to clarify initially is whether your position falls under the global billing Medicare/Medicaid exempt category. If your position is classified as Medicare exempt, you will be unable to bill for any services. You should be able to determine this from discussion with someone in your human resources department. If you are not exempt and thus eligible to bill, you will also need to understand the rules surrounding the daily concurrent hospital billing done by the various providers.

KEEPING TRACK OF PRODUCTIVITY

When you begin to plan for billing for professional CNS services, it is extremely helpful to sit down with two people in your organization: your immediate supervisor and the person who will be submitting your billing statements. The latter is usually a certified coder. Developing a good working relationship with a coder can be of tremendous value as you embark on this learning expedition. The coder will have extensive knowledge of reimbursement, documentation requirements, and coding, and can be one of your best resources for questions. Networking with other CNSs in your organization who are already recognized Medicare providers can facilitate the process of learning and save you time and frustration as well. I also recommend that you discuss up front with your supervisor how the revenue generated by the services you provide will be handled. In some agreements, reimbursement for CNS services goes directly into the company and is considered a way of offsetting your salary. This seems, in my experience, to be the most common practice. You may want to negotiate some type of productivity bonus that you receive when a certain level of productivity is achieved. Another recommendation is to create some sort of tracking mechanism that will allow you to see how you are spending your time. For example, if your practice encompasses both hospital visits and clinic or office follow-up visits, you would want to be able to see where your time is spent and what level and types of services you are providing. You should be able to receive monthly printouts showing the volume of hospital follow-up visits, admissions, discharges, consults, and any procedures, as well as the dollar amounts billed for each service. The reimbursement allowed for each service will vary somewhat from year to year as well and is determined by the PFS, which is updated annually. Reimbursement amounts also depend on the individual third-party payer, with Medicare being one of the lowest payers. You will also want to know the average collection rate for services billed. This is another area where your billing person can come in handy. Depending on the type of practice you are in and the volume of physician services you provide, you may be amazed at the financial contribution you are making to an organization.

SUMMARY

Although the rules and regulations of the reimbursement process can be overwhelming, it is important that the CNS has a good understanding of the regulations, terminology, and legalities surrounding reimbursement.

Resources such as coding and billing seminars and conferences, independent study programs, continuing education programs, journal articles, and coding and billing experts are available and can provide valuable assistance. Sitting down with other CNSs who have already "mastered" the reimbursement puzzle can be invaluable. I say "mastered" in jest because in my experience it is an ongoing learning experience. Visit the government website for the Centers for Medicare and Medicaid Services to obtain firsthand, up-to-date information. Your goal should be to understand current guidelines, requirements for accurate documentation of E/M codes, rules, regulations, and laws that govern you as a provider in your state to minimize your risk of fraudulent claims. Because of the dynamic nature of the reimbursement landscape, the CNS should be aware of these resources for billing and reimbursement and seek them out as opportunities for demonstrating the financial contributions of the CNS that will undoubtedly continue to grow.

One last consideration for the CNS who bills is the increase in liability incurred. A well-intentioned provider can commit billing fraud if poorly informed. Even if your organization has a billing and coding department that actually prepares and submits the bill, you are accountable for knowing the rules and requirements for documentation for reimbursement. Prepare yourself by taking advantage of courses designed to help you learn and maintain current knowledge about billing rules and regulations. Additionally, you will need to ensure that you carry adequate liability insurance.

Billing and reimbursement issues may seem overwhelming at first, and are certainly challenging, but they can be fun and rewarding, too.

REFERENCES

Baker, J. J., & Baker, R. W. (2014). *Health care finance: Basic tools for nonfinancial managers* (4th ed.). Dallas, TX: Jones & Bartlett Learning.

Balanced Budget Act of 1997. (1997). United States Public Law 105-33: Subtitle F; Chapter 1-Services of Health Professionals; Subchapter B-Other Healthcare Professionals, Section 4511; August 5, 1997.

Baradell, J., & Hanrahan, N. (2000). CPT coding and medicare reimbursement issues. *Clinical Nurse Specialist, 14*(6), 299–303.

Bendix, J. (2013). Cracking the code: Top strategies for selecting appropriate E/M levels and documenting patient care. *Medical Economics, 90*(10), 20–25.

Brassard, A. (2015). APRN policy and payment. *Nurse Leader, 13*(2), 36–38.

Centers for Medicare and Medicaid Services. (2014a). *Medicare benefit policy manual: Covered medical and other health services.* Publication 100-02. Retrieved from http://www.cms.gov/Regulations-and-Guidance/Guidance/Manuals/Internet-Only-Manuals-IOMs-Items/CMS012673.html

Centers for Medicare and Medicaid Services. (2014b). *Medicare program integrity manual: Covered medical and other health services.* Medicare Enrollment Publication 100-08. Retrieved from www.cms.gov/regulations-and-guidance/guidance/manuals/internet-only-manuals-IOMs-Items/CMS012673.html

Centers for Medicare and Medicaid Services. (2015). *Medicare information for advanced practice registered nurses, anesthesiologist assistants and physician assistants.* Retrieved from http://cms.gov/outreach-and-education/Medicare-Learning-Network-MLN/MLNProducts/Downloads/Medicare-Information-for-APRNs

Chapman, S. A., Wides, C. D., & Spetz, J. (2010). Payment regulations for advanced practice nurses: Implications for primary care. *Policy, Politics, & Nursing Practice, 11*(2), 89–98.

Craig, D. J. (2014). Maximizing reimbursement: What nurse practitioners need to know. *Nurse Practitioner, 39*(8), 16–18.

Dowling, R. (2014). Incident-to billing: Your questions answered. *Medical Economics, 91*(16), 50.

Gapenski, L. C. (2012). *Fundamentals of healthcare finance* (2nd ed.). Chicago, IL: Health Administration Press. Retrieved from https://www.ache.org/pubs/gapenski_chapter3.pdf

Gray, L. (2014). ICD-10: Time to take action. *Medical Economics, 91*(7), 36–39.

Richmond, T. S., Thompson, H. J., & Sullivan-Marx, E. M. (2000). Reimbursement for acute care nurse practitioner services. *American Journal of Critical Care, 9*(1), 52–61.

Zuzelo, P. R., Fallon, R., Lang, C., & Mount, L. (2004). Clinical nurse specialists' knowledge specific to Medicare structures and processes. *Clinical Nurse Specialist, 18*(4), 207–217.

CHAPTER 24

Starting Collaborative Practice With Physicians or Clinics: What You Should Know

CAROL L. DELVILLE
SHERI INNERARITY
GLENDA JOINER-ROGERS

Today's practice environment for the clinical nurse specialist (CNS) in the United States is in a dynamic state with critical elements that influence the ways advanced practice registered nurses (APRNs) are recognized and regulated, varying between the federal-level and state-to-state rules and regulations. A large part of the confusion is related to differences in how federal and state legislation and regulations and professional organizations define the terms "independent practice," "collaborative practice," "delegated practice," and "supervised practice." The confusion is further complicated by the lack of consistency in how CNS practice is recognized and utilized within states. This chapter presents an overview of current practice definitions and refers you to resources where you will be able to find updated information regarding legislative changes that transform the practice environment. Key issues for establishing a collaborative practice are presented, including elements within a practice agreement, obtaining hospital credentialing, defining the protocols for practice, and ensuring that a practice is adequately reviewed and meets quality and safety standards. Salary and practice payment structures are presented to aid in the critical initial practice contracts decision-making process.

PRACTICE TYPES

Independent Practice

The term "independent practitioner" originated with The Joint Commission for purposes of credentialing and clinical privileges, and is used for this purpose by the U.S. Health Resources and Human Services Administration

(Health Resources and Services Administration [HRSA], 2014; Department of Health and Human Services [DHHS], 2014). The Joint Commission (2015) defines an independent practitioner as "an individual, as permitted by law and regulation, and by the organization, to provide care and services, without direction or supervision, within the scope of the individual's license and consistent with the privileges granted by the organization." Why does this matter? Decisions on who may perform admission history and physical exams, order restraints, work in federally supported health centers, or who is required to be credentialed in hospitals are all based on how the term "licensed independent practitioner" is defined by the regulators (Centers for Medicare and Medicaid [CMS] and HRSA), accreditors (The Joint Commission), and individual state rules and regulations (CMS, 2014; HRSA, 2015).

The National Council of State Boards of Nursing (NCSBN) defines independent practice as "no required written collaborative agreement, no supervision, no conditions to practice" (NCSBN, 2015). The NCSBN reported that as of March 2015, CNS practice is recognized as "independent" in 24 states plus the District of Columbia, and the Commonwealth of Northern Mariana Islands, with 15 of those states and the District of Columbia permitting independent prescribing. The NCSBN maintains up-to-date state maps on state recognition of CNS practice as independent, not independent, or no advanced practice authority (NCSBN, 2015). Given these definitions, "independent practitioner" does not need to mean that a CNS is practicing in isolation. CMS reimbursement is based on an individual's national provider identifier (NPI) and is paid directly to the physician or "nonphysician provider" (Form CMS-855I) or to a clinic or group practice (Form CMS-855B) depending on the structure of the practice agreement (DHHS, 2014). The CMS considers the CNS an independent provider or fee-for-service contractor when making direct payments. A CNS may bill the CMS independently (e.g., as a diabetic educator), under the individual's NPI (i.e., as an independent practitioner), or in those states where the CNS is authorized to provide "physician services" with direct billing to insurance, Medicare, or Medicaid (CMS, 2014). However, a CNS in a delegated, collaborative, or supervised practice may be required to submit CMS billing as "incident to" under the physician's NPI number (DHHS, 2014).

Supervised Versus Delegated Practice

Physician supervision of CNS practice is required in some settings (e.g., nursing homes) by the Omnibus Reconciliation Act of 1987 and CMS guidelines (CMS, 2014). Supervision is considered to have three components: (a) administrative; (b) educational; and (c) supportive (American Medical Director Association [AMDA] Ad Hoc Work Group, 2011). Supervision is often viewed in a hierarchical context, with the expectation that the relationship will mature into a collaborative practice as trust is built over time. Theoretically, the ultimate goal of supervision is patient safety. Supervision should focus on competency (the ability to comprehend, elaborate, and apply knowledge to a required task or skill performance) and responsibility (management of tasks without direct one-on-one supervision within the accepted CNS scope of practice). This requires a clear delineation of role and practice expectations by both the supervising physician and the CNS. For example, when working with a client with diabetes, it is essential to have clearly identified which practice guideline(s) is to be used for a client in an acute versus a long-term care setting. Several states have rules and regulations requiring scheduled supervision, often stepwise, with more frequent supervision in new practice relationships (AMDA Ad Hoc Work Group, 2011).

Delegation (of duties) or the ability to perform "medical acts" is a state regulatory term describing the supervisory relationship in which medical care is delegated to another person, such as an APRN. Delegated acts are defined by the states, and may require direct physician supervision (in person, or in some cases via telehealth, radio, etc.). Responsibility for the delegation outside of the CNS scope of practice varies with state rules and regulations. One example of a delegated medical act is the ability to prescribe either medication or durable medical equipment. The CNS may be required to include the physician's identification and/or varying levels of supervision of prescriptions written. As of March 2015, CNSs have independent prescribing in 16 states, the District of Columbia, and the Commonwealth of Northern Mariana Islands. A CNS has "no independent prescribing," meaning collaborative or delegated prescribing in an additional 18 states and the Virgin Islands, permitting the CNS the ability to prescribe in a total of 35 U.S. states, districts, or territories (NCSBN, 2015).

Collaborative Practice

Collaborative practice is a dynamic, interpersonal process allowing two or more individuals an opportunity to make a commitment to interact and constructively solve problems, learn from each other, and jointly identify goals and outcome objectives (Hamric, Hanson, Tracy, & O'Grady, 2014). The benefits for the collaborative team are considerable and include increased productivity, time, decreased redundancy of care, shared expertise, and promotion of trust and respect between professions. As with the term "independent practitioner," collaborative practice has a number of different definitions stemming from practice models, Medicare regulation, the Social Security Act, and national medical and nursing associations and state guidelines. The most common definition for collaborative practice is "a joint cooperative arrangement that integrates individual expertise between the individual team members" (AMDA Ad Hoc Working Group, 2011). This definition recognizes the unique and diverse knowledge contributed by each member of the health care team. An extensive review of federal, professional organizations, and select experts defining collaboration illustrates a diverse perspective ranging from "delegation" (42 CFR 483.40 e) to the "ongoing interdisciplinary communication regarding the care of individuals and populations of patients in order to promote care" (American College of Physicians; www.amda.com/advocacy/ReviewDefinitions.pdf). Collaborative practice at its best recognizes the differences in perspective that each member contributes to the health care team. The NCSBN (2015) position is that collaborative practice should be the "professional norm" and recognizes that no single professional activity defines a profession.

PRACTICE AGREEMENTS

While it is difficult to keep up with legislative changes in CNS practice in the United States, many states require collaborative, delegated, or supervised medical practice. Currently, 41 states allow CNSs to practice either independently or with some variation of a practice agreement. Thus, state regulatory requirements form the basis for many decisions related to practice, and the perception of whether working is independent or delegated, collaborative or supervised.

Credentialing

Credentialing is required for facility-based practice, such as a hospital, and also to join insurance provider panels. The basics of credentialing involve being recognized by the board of nursing in the state of practice. The minimum requirements, as of 2015, include a registered nursing license; minimum of a master's degree in advanced practice nursing (or completion of a post-master's certificate program); passing a credentialing exam, usually the American Nurses Credentialing Center (ANCC) or American Association of Critical-Care Nurses Certification Corporation (AACN); and submission of all required documents to the relevant board. Maintaining CNS certification requires a minimum of 400 practice hours every 5 years, and a minimum of 75 continuing education (CE) contact hours (25 hours in pharmacology) as half of the professional development for license renewal. The remaining half of professional development hours may be completed by any combination of six professional development categories: CE hours, academic credit, presentations, preceptor for an APRN graduate student, publication or research, or professional service (ANCC, 2015). It is imperative that the APRN maintain a current file of relevant materials.

Credentialing is entirely another step and can be onerous to say the least. Some facilities require the APRN to have an NPI, Department of Public Safety (DPS; e.g., Texas) and Drug Enforcement Agency (DEA) licenses, whether or not they need to prescribe medications/controlled substances. In states where delegated/collaborative/supervised physician practice is required, the APRN will need to provide a written practice agreement (WPA) between the APRN and relevant physician(s).

Facilities may also require a Basic Life Support certificate or Advanced Life Support certificate, depending on the population with which one works. Generally clinic practices do not require all of these documents for practice as an APRN; however, billing insurance companies requires credentialing to be listed as a provider on the insurance provider panel, so as more APRNs obtain independent practice, more APRNs will need these basic credentialing documents.

Credentialing also requires letters of reference/completed standardized reference forms. Most faculty fill out these forms for recent graduates, and even for some graduates who have been practicing for years, but who are functioning as preceptors. Since being credentialed involves being "recredentialed," much of this process is a recurring responsibility for the APRN. Keeping a file with all current materials is vital, as the APRN may be audited by the state licensing board or credentialing bodies. In some facilities, ongoing evaluations are required of the APRN to remain credentialed.

Protocols

Protocols have many different definitions, but for the purposes of this chapter "formal ideas, plans, or expectations concerning the actions of those involved in patient care..." (Venes, 2009, p. 1916) will suffice. Protocols may be part of a practice agreement between an APRN and physicians, and typically functions as a "recipe" for practice related to specific diagnoses. The CMS requires clinics to provide a protocol for practice in clinics accepting Medicare and Medicaid patients. In relation to the CMS requirements, these can be as simple as an agreement to use F. Domino's (current edition) *Five Minute Clinical Consult*, or an agreement to use *Epocrates©* as a basis for the standard of patient care.

When creating a WPA, prescriptive authority agreement (PAA), or collaborative agreement, the "cookbook" method of using a text is often not required, or included in the written document. At a minimum, an agreement of this type needs to have the full names and credentials, including all license numbers, scope of practice credentials, as well as the NPI, DPS, and DEA numbers. There is usually a description of the scope of practice involved; for example, a pediatric nurse practitioner (PNP) will not see any patient older than the age of 18 (or whatever is negotiated).

In some states, such as currently in Texas, the PAA must include what medications may or may not be prescribed. While it is onerous to list *all* the medications that may be prescribed, it's somewhat easier to list classes of medications that the APRN won't prescribe; for example: "The APRN will not prescribe chemotherapy." Regardless, this needs to be agreed upon and signed, in those states in which it is required, prior to any evaluation and management of patients by the APRN. If the APRN will be working with more than one physician, all relevant provider credentials need to be part of the practice agreement, as well as signature(s) to the document. An annual review of the WPA or PAA and resigning by all involved parties are required. Some states may require the delegation/collaboration/agreement to be registered with the board of medicine. This may be required for *every physician* with whom the APRN works. If the APRN is in a large practice, this may involve many physicians. In a facility-based practice, the chief of staff using a generic practice agreement may meet this requirement.

Some physicians (e.g., specialists) may also want to have separate written agreements with APRNs delineating or specifying the APRN practice. Settings with a very limited scope of practice, such as Planned Parenthood, might even have a more restrictive practice agreement, with specific classes of medications that may be prescribed delineated in the practice agreement.

Quality Assurance and Peer Review

In states requiring a practice agreement, there is often a requirement for a quality improvement, practice improvement, or peer review. CMS requires a quarterly meeting of the peer review committee to review records of all providers, not just the APRN's patient records. Many practice agreements require either record review or face-to-face meetings regarding patient care. Some states still require physician supervision a certain number of days monthly, or a record review of a percentage of patient records periodically. With telemedicine easily available, APRNs and physicians can Skype or use Facetime on cell phones to communicate regarding patient care. There are many types of quality assurance documents available online that may be downloaded and used to set the standard of care for a variety of diagnoses (Romano, Hussy, & Ritley, 2010). It is often simplest to utilize a textbook that is reviewed annually, such as Domino's *Five Minute Clinical Consult*, as a protocol, cookbook, or standard of care for quality assurance. Each diagnosis in Domino's text is written and reviewed annually by an expert in that field.

Another method to consider for quality assurance is regular referral to specialists, or other physicians, which can be very useful in complex patients. In fact, CMS has a requirement that new patients are to be seen by the physician, who is to develop the plan of care, and afterward, the APRN may see the patient. This is not a requirement of most insurance companies. The Agency for Healthcare Research and Quality (AHRQ) has several resources available for providers to improve practice and patient safety retrievable from http://www .ahrq.gov/professionals/quality-patient-safety/quality-resources/tools/office-testing-toolkit/index.html.

REIMBURSEMENT

The CNS working in a collaborative practice receives compensation for services in a variety of ways including salary, subcontracting, Medicare, Medicaid, and other third-party insurance companies, concierge model of medical care, and private pay. The following paragraphs discuss each of these payment mechanisms for the CNS.

Salary Versus Subcontracting

A salaried position offers the CNS a constant revenue source, which is advantageous to the CNS who is new to an organization or practice. Many salaried positions specify the number of patient encounters the CNS is expected to manage within a day. Depending on the practice, visits may be short and focused, with 15 to 20 minutes for established patients, or as long as an hour for a new patient with multiple complex medical conditions. It is not unusual for a CNS new to the practice, especially a new CNS graduate, to have a reduced patient load initially (perhaps the first few months in the practice) until the office routine and patient cases become familiar. A salaried position affords the CNS an opportunity to maintain a revenue source until he or she can work up to a full caseload and see a specified number of patients in the allotted time frame designated by the practice. In addition to the generation of revenue created by the CNS seeing patients and billing for "physician services," the CNS may develop programs that result in cost savings and thus increases to the practice revenue. There should be a means to reflect how this performance will result in an increase and/or bonus to the CNS's salary. It is advisable to have performance measures (caseloads, revenue generation, quality outcomes, etc.) clearly identified in the practice agreement. Benefits are an additional source of income for a salaried position, which should be negotiated by the CNS to include compensation for health care, vacation, continuing education, malpractice insurance, an equipment budget, as well as time for mentorship and supervision (Beauvais, 2016).

The CNS who works in a subcontracted position collaborates with a physician or physician group practice to manage the care of patients. Depending in which state the CNS practices, the physician(s) may provide additional services to the CNS including chart review, collaboration/consultation, and/or prescriptive authority delegation (Hamric et al., 2014). In return for access to the patients and these physician services, the CNS negotiates payment to the physician(s) based on a percentage of the CNS's reimbursement for "physician services." Physician services is a term used by Medicare (as well as other third-party payers) to directly reimburse the CNS when he or she performs what are considered to be physician services or those services which would be physician services if furnished by a physician (Balanced Budget Act, 1997). Currently, Medicare services are directly reimbursed to the CNS at 85% of the physician fee schedule (CMS, 2014). This negotiated payment agreement should be included in the practice agreement and, if required, a contractual agreement between the CNS and the physician or physician group practice.

An important decision for any CNS in a salaried or subcontracted position will be to consider whether he or she will attempt the complicated and constantly changing process of medical billing and perform self-billing of "physician services," or hire a professional medical billing service with experience in medical billing. Revenue stability for the CNS and physician practice is based on timely submission of "physician services" and resubmission of any rejected payments. The CNS may well not have the time or opportunity to participate in self-billing of services since the CNS will already be involved in the provision of "physician services" for the patient, as well as completion of the patient clinical encounter and documentation of the encounter in the patient's medical record, and will often complete the patient's bill for services. If the CNS chooses to use the professional medical billing service, the CNS must be closely involved in the actual payment collection from the patient or third-party payer (Hamric et al., 2014).

Medicare/Medicaid Versus Insurance Reimbursement

Medicare, Medicaid, and insurance carriers are considered third-party payers and are the primary sources along with private pay that reimburse the CNS for "physician services" during a patient clinical encounter. The CNS in a salaried or subcontracted position who provides "physician services" to patients whose health care is covered by Medicare, Medicaid, or private insurance companies, does so using Current Procedural Terminology (CPT) codes and International Classification of Diseases (ICD) ICD-9, or as of October 2015, ICD-10 codes. The CPT codes that are assigned to "physician services" rendered must represent the level of evaluation and management (E/M) services performed. E/M services include the extent of history obtained, the extent of the physical examination, and the complexity of the medical decision making, which must be accompanied by documentation of the level of care provided and billed. The CPT and E/M codes are used universally in determining reimbursement to the provider from Medicare, Medicaid, insurance companies, and other third-party payers (Hamric et al., 2014).

The CNS can and should use the payments received from the third-party payer, private pay, and any other sources of payment or revenue generation for the practice, to estimate and evaluate his or her value to the practice. This information provides clear evidence for the CNS to use in negotiations for an increase in salary and bonuses when expectations, such as an increase in the growth of the business and revenue, are exceeded. Further, the subcontracting CNS may also negotiate for a decrease in percentage of payment to the collaborating physician/practice when revenues goals, savings to the practice, quality improvements, and other expectations are exceeded.

Concierge Medicine Versus Private Pay

In today's health care market, some practices have switched to alternative billing methods other than traditional third-party payers and private insurance carriers. Concierge medicine refers to a wide variety of nontraditional models in which a limited number of patients pay a fixed fee monthly or annually for enhanced services including more time spent with patients, greater one-on-one interaction, and improved provider access after hours. These services are often noncovered services in the traditional third-party payer model. Concierge medicine may or may not offer billing to third-party payers and insurance carriers for "physician services" (Ahmed, 2015). In concierge medicine, the patient-to-provider ratio is kept small to provide more time and personalized care, thus patient satisfaction is a key outcome.

In private pay, the patient pays for all physician services as care is accessed. Typically there are price list structures for every service provided to the client. Many options may be developed based on the patient's ability to pay or some amount less than what would be received if "physician services" were billed. In essence, concierge medicine and private pay medicine save money and subsequently increase revenue for the practice by eliminating overhead billing costs (Ahmed, 2015).

The CNS who works in a collaborative practice that utilizes a concierge model of payment for services and/or accepts private payment for patient services should develop a plan for reimbursement of the CNS's services for these patients when the CNS begins employment in the collaborative practice. Given that billing costs are usually eliminated with both methods of payment, there may be an opportunity for the CNS to have a greater amount of income for these patient clinical encounters.

SUMMARY

The initial steps for a CNS to establish when entering any new collaborative practice arrangement with a physician or clinic are to clearly define the type of practice relationship (independent, collaborative, supervisory, delegated, etc.), billing methods utilized by the practice, and how the CNS's reimbursement will be calculated based on caseload and job performance. With the consensus model helping to align educational requirements for licensure across states, and the Institute of Medicine's report on the future of nursing advocating for APRNs to function "to the full extent of their education," there will continue to be changes in federal and state rules and regulations, creating confusion for all parties entering contract negotiations (NCSBN, 2015). Having current and accurate information regarding CNS rules and regulations and knowing how to negotiate a practice agreement that reflects the scope of CNS practice permitted by federal, state, and credentialing bodies (facilities and hospitals) are a professional and legal responsibility.

On a final note, there are many other details to consider when entering into a collaborative practice contractual agreement. Consider the duration of the contract and if there is a "no compete clause" meaning the CNS will be restricted from working in the area or field for a designated period of time if he or she leaves the practice. Specify under what circumstances the CNS's contract can be terminated. For example, will the CNS's termination be based on the CNS's performance and, if so, who will conduct the performance evaluation? Be clear if severance can be based on financial considerations should the CNS or the physician have a better job offer. Clearly identify how much notice is required when either the CNS or physician wants to leave the practice. Will there be on-call responsibilities for the CNS? If the answer is yes, how will on-call be managed—by phone or is there 24/7 provider access in the practice? Although there are many resources available to help the CNS with contract negotiation, consider having a legal professional review any contract prior to finalizing the arrangement. Obtaining a legal opinion or contract review will assist the CNS to clearly understand the contractual agreement and will provide the opportunity to clarify any concerns before signing the contract.

REFERENCES

Ahmed, H. (2015). Cash-only and concierge-based medicine: Roles in the health care payment landscape. *Harvard Medical Student Review*. Retrieved from http://www.hmsreview.org/?article=cash-concierge-based-medicine-roles-health-care-payment-landscape

American Medical Director Association Ad Hoc Work Group on the Role of the Attending Physician and Advanced Practice Nurse. (2011). Collaborative and supervisory relationships between attending physicians and advanced practice nurses in long-term care facilities. *Geriatric Nursing, 32*(1), 7–17. Retrieved from http://ac.elscdn.com.ezproxy.lib.utexas.edu/S0197457210005562/1-s2.0-S0197457210005562-main.pdf?_tid=a7d1e64c-cd8b-11e4-896e00000aab0f01&acdnat=1426696222_2b54a86b03c79c94acd43b5c5e26809e

American Nurses Credentialing Center. (2015). *2015 certification renewal requirements.* Retrieved from http://www.nursecredentialing.org/RenewalRequirements.aspx

Balanced Budget Act of 1997. (1997). United States Public Law 105-33: Subtitle F; Chapter 1-Services of Health Professionals; Subchapter B-Other Healthcare Professionals, Section 4511: August 5, 1997.

Beauvais. A. (2016). Role transition: Strategies for success in the marketplace. In S. M. Denisco & A. M. Barker (Eds.), *Advanced practice nursing* (3rd ed.). Burlington, VT: Jones and Bartlett Learning.

Department of Health and Human Services. (2014). *Centers for Medicare and Medicaid Services. CMS manual system.* Pub. 100-07 State Operations. Retrieved from http://www.cms.gov/Regulations-and-Guidance/Guidance/Manuals/Internet-Only-Manuals-IOMs-Items/CMS1201984.html

Hamric, A. B., Hanson, C. M., Tracy, M. F., & O'Grady, E. T. (Eds.). (2014). *Advanced nursing practice: An integrated approach* (5th ed.). St. Louis, MO: Elsevier.

Health Resources and Services Administration. (2014). *Primary care: The health center program. Clarification of credentialing and privileging policy.* Retrieved from http://bphc.hrsa.gov/policiesregulations/policies/pdfs/pin200222.pdf

Joint Commission on Accreditation of Healthcare Organizations. (2015). *2015 comprehensive accreditation manual for hospitals.* Oakbridge, IL: Joint Commission.

National Council of State Boards of Nursing. (2015). Retrieved from National Council of State Boards of Nursing website pages: https://www.ncsbn.org/index.htm, https://www.ncsbn.org/5406.htm, https://www.ncsbn.org/738.htm, and https://www.ncsbn.org/5410.htm

Romano, P. S., Hussy, P., & Ritley, D. (2010). *Selecting quality and resource use measures: A decision guide for community collaboratives.* Rockville, MD: Agency for Healthcare Research and Quality. AHRQ publication No. 09(10)-0073.

Venes, D. (2009). *Taber's cyclopedic medical dictionary* (21st ed.). Philadelphia, PA: F.A. Davis.

CHAPTER 25

Secrets for a Joyful Life as a Clinical Nurse Specialist

JANET S. FULTON

The purpose of this book is to offer some practical advice and considered perspectives about the clinical nurse specialist (CNS) role for those beginning their career journey as CNSs. It is now my task in this final chapter to integrate the ideas and offer some parting thoughts. I decided to revisit the sage advice of Dr. Grayce Sills, Professor Emeritus, The Ohio State University, College of Nursing, originally shared in a 1986 commencement address to graduates of the Miami Valley School of Nursing in Dayton, Ohio, on the occasion of the closing of the diploma school. The address helped finalize an era and launch the future (Sills, 1986). A new CNS is in much the same position, leaving one period of a career behind while launching a new direction. Dr. Sills offered the new graduates seven secrets for a joyful life in nursing. This chapter revisits those seven secrets, updated and reconsidered, for beginning a CNS career: life-long learning, collaboration, creative deviance, investment in the profession, families and communities, appreciation of difference, and humor.

LIFE-LONG LEARNING

Life-long learning is a commitment to curiosity. Approach each day with curiosity and develop the art of asking good questions. Good questions are more important than correct answers. Could American ingenuity have landed a man on the moon and brought him back again unless someone first asked the question "Can we go to the moon and back?" Forward direction is initiated by thoughtful, adventurous questions asked by really curious thinkers.

Knowledge serves to shape questions and provoke possibilities. Ideas come from the intellectual work of asking questions, envisioning possibilities, and juxtaposing unrelated notions. Knowledge is expanding at rates that no one could have ever predicted. Life-long learning has moved beyond reading journals and attending professional conferences. While journals and conferences remain important, physical access to information is omnipresent electronically, thanks largely to the Internet and "smart" personal devices. Life-long learning is now more about being a savvy evaluator of information than a person with a good memory for details.

New CNSs should search for ideas in the most unlikely of places. The electronic information age requires only a mouse click or screen touch to find a new perspective. Constantly ask questions about the reliability of information. Not all information may be reliable, but should it be summarily dismissed? Consider the implications.

Information from the Web can help broaden your perspective, as in "who knew" that was even a consideration. For example: An undergraduate student, observing ketamine being used clinically, decided to write a paper about nursing care of patients receiving the drug. Searching the Internet she found websites that provided instructions for abuse of the drug and testimonials to the benefits of illegal use, whereupon she added a section to her paper about the drug's potential for abuse. If her search had been limited to professional journals, her information, and surely her perspective, would have been more limited.

COLLABORATION

Life is a group project. Our very existence in a complex society requires collaboration. Health care settings are highly complex systems where people's lives literally depend on the ability of the workers in the system to collaborate for common purpose. No doubt your CNS course work included content on collaboration in a multidisciplinary environment. Collaboration is a fundamental competency that should become second nature for any CNS. Invest early and often in collaborative relationships—they will return a thousand-fold!

Extend the idea of collaboration beyond the *interdisciplinary health care team*. Consider the contributions of employees working in areas such as maintenance, supply services, housekeeping, parking, and the gift shop. Coworkers in these ancillary areas make critical contributions to the environment in which we practice. Flip the switch and the light goes on; fill the trash can, and it gets emptied; food trays are sterilized, drapes vacuumed, snow removed in winter. Consider what would happen if these workers were not part of the *environmental team*.

In our daily work it is all too easy to get caught up in the invidious distinctions that divide us, cautioned Dr. Sills. It is good to remember the value that unites us—each of us desires the best possible end and the highest possible good for those we serve. Assume each person is working to the best of his or her ability. Commitment to teamwork means asking, "How can I help you?"

The health care environment is a microcosm of society. It includes highly educated professionals with prestige and social privilege working alongside persons with no professional credential or minimum education. We serve a common purpose—work collaboratively, everyone included. The team is bigger than you think and your success is dependent on many others you don't see.

Collaborate within the professional community. Engage CNSs in other specialty areas, in other health care systems, and in the greater community of similar interests. Many a project starts out with a burst of energy only to languish as work seems to drag and enthusiasm fades. Collaborating with others helps provide needed support and energy that will see the project to completion. Be a colleague; have a colleague.

CREATIVE DEVIANCE

Deviance is behavior that is sharply different from customary or traditional and is, in itself, value neutral. A CNS is, by design, a deviant nurse—someone who thinks and acts differently. Embrace difference and wear it comfortably. Creative deviance is the source of innovation. Nurture your creativity by asking every day what can be done to improve quality, decrease cost, and enhance safety for patients and staff. How to do it differently and better!

Creative deviance is contagious; be sure to infect the staff. Ask "I wonder if ..." rhetorical questions in staff forums and committee meetings. Cultivate a climate of curiosity, and over time measure success by the number of new ideas that come from the staff. A staff nurse once asked my opinion about two methods for drawing blood from a central line. I asked her what she considered to be the better method. She replied that in all her years of nursing, no one had ever asked her opinion. How sad, and yet what an opportunity! As a result of her initial inquiry, the procedure was changed. Creative deviance will flourish when staff are empowered.

Be kind and considerate, but persistent, as others will sometimes find your deviant thinking slightly irritating. Learn to read the rhythm of the situation, the ebb and flow of daily work demands, and group dynamics. But don't wait for consensus. While waiting for agreement, the window of opportunity may close. Consensus can also be a tyrant demanding agreement in situations where difference should be encouraged. Nursing has a convention of conformity, dating to our early history in military and religious traditions. Avoid the tyranny of consensus. Empower yourself to move ideas forward.

INVESTMENT IN THE PROFESSION

As a nurse with a graduate degree, you are one of few in a profession of many and an ambassador for the CNS role. Join professional organizations and give back to the profession by being an active contributor. Serve on committees and in leadership positions. Find a mentor; be a mentor. Many volunteer hours have been donated by others to move the profession forward. It takes the collective energy of professional organizations to make an impact. Commit time and energy to advancing the profession.

In addition, give your treasure, too. It's important to give back by paying professional organizational dues and donating money to professional foundations. Contributions to foundations are essential for supporting nursing scholarships and research. Give back to your school. It's highly likely that somewhere along your career path you were helped by someone who gave back. It's your profession—invest in its future.

FAMILIES AND COMMUNITIES

Keep family first. Dr. Sills reminds us that family is where your spirit resides, where you are nourished and loved. Family protects and defends. Family renews. Your health is intricately woven in the fabric of your family. Your health is family health.

Your family members supported your education; they sacrificed your time and attention in exchange for classes and course work. Your family believes in you. Value your family's support by striving always to be the best that you can be.

Invest in your community. Communities are the harbingers of health values. Be aware of local issues that have health implications, and be informed about prevailing political sentiments, controversial issues, and the pros and cons associated with civic issues. Interact with others around common interests. Parents know that children's activities generate opportunities to be present, such as at sporting events, music recitals, and school fundraising programs. Other opportunities include civic associations and volunteering. Your presence as a parent/volunteer brings an advanced nursing perspective to your community where you can influence others for a healthy community. Contribute to the community newspaper a health article in your area of specialty. Together with your local CNS network, create a list of specialty experts whom local media can contact for commentary and informational contributions. Host an "Ask a Nurse" column in the local newspaper, radio show, or civic website. Health and safety issues are embedded in many public policies. Support legislation that advances health. Meet with your local and state legislators; they need to know you and have you on their contact list when expert health opinions are needed. Think about health and safety implications when communities deal with issues such as food labeling, bike helmet laws, and immunization requirements. As a leader in nursing, seek to influence the public welfare. Local politics is a perfect place to invest in the health of your community.

APPRECIATION OF DIFFERENCE

On a grand scale the world is shrinking every day, not literally in size, of course, but obstacles to human communication and interaction are disappearing. No longer is physical travel required to work with others. We connect, communicate, and work virtually, coming together around a topic of mutual interest for a common purpose. No more working in silos divided by profession, employment, country, or continent. Think globally; work globally; influence globally!

Our natural tendency is to fear that which is different. Childhood experiences create our sense of familiar and we are all most comfortable in our own nests. That which is different is subject to suspicion, discrimination, petty meanness, and forgone conclusions—ways of thinking that will erode a CNS's ability to lead. Strive to be amicable and approachable, because the ability to influence others depends on their perceiving your acceptance of their difference. And remember, you are the "different other" in their eyes. Respect differences and look for common ground.

HUMOR

Take your work seriously and yourself lightly. Humor is found in recognizing oddities and inconsistencies in a situation, and the daily work of patient care in a complex system provides more than enough opportunity for humor. The ability to grin in the face of the bizarre and to laugh at incongruence brings energy and renewal to both stiflingly boring tasks and epochs of human tragedy.

The well-known comedian George Carlin was a master at finding humor in incongruence. Here are some examples from his book *Brain Droppings* (Carlin, 1997):

- Every time you use the phrase "all my life" it has a different meaning. (p. 194)
- How is it possible to be seated on a standing committee? (p. 195)
- I put a dollar in one of those change machines. Nothing changed. (p. 197)

Look for humor; find joy. Every day comes with its own surprises.

Of course, not every day will be full of joy, but each day can be a joyful adventure in your personal pursuit of excellence. Go forward in your new CNS career and make each day a new opportunity by pursuing curiosities and striving for excellence. I'll end this chapter with the same quote Dr. Sills used to end her commencement address. Though dated in its publication, it is timeless in sentiment:

A profession should make us more human, not less so; more alive, not less so; more dedicated, not less so; and we default on our professional birthright unless we can reach out to others and communicate this feeling of concern for the common bond between all of us. It is the food upon which your spirit feeds. It is the sustenance that helps motivate your patients to get well, or, rather, your fellow human to get well. You must give them this above all, and you must try even when they seem unable to accept it or profit by it. We fail others when we fail ourselves and when we succeed with ourselves we inevitably succeed with others (Whitehouse, 1962).

REFERENCES

Carlin, G. (1997). *Brain droppings*. New York, NY: Hyperion.

Sills, G. M. (1986). *The quest for excellence: The joy of nursing*. Paper presented at the Eighty-eighth Commencement, Miami Valley Hospital School of Nursing, Dayton, OH.

Whitehouse, F. A. (1962). The rationale of nursing. *Rehabilitation Record, 3*(4), 12.

Index

Accreditation Association for the
Ambulatory Healthcare
(AAAHC), 211
acute care clinical nurse specialist
(CNS), 182
ad hoc group, 88
Adult-Gerontology Clinical Nurse
Specialist–Board Certified
(AGCNS-BC), 206
Advanced Life Support certificate, 230
advanced oncology clinical nurse
specialist (AOCNS), 204
advanced practice registered nurses
(APRNs), 15, 29, 215
Advanced Practice Registered Nurse
(APRN) Consensus Model, 5, 16
Affordable Care Act, 23, 157
Agency for Healthcare Research and
Quality (AHRQ), 232
agreements, practice
credentialing, 230–231
protocols, 231
quality assurance and
peer review, 232
AHRQ. *See* Agency for Healthcare
Research and Quality
American Association of Critical Care
Nurses Certification Corporation
(AACN cert. corp.), 204
American Board of Nursing Specialties
(ABNS) certification, 204
American Nurses Association (ANA)
credentialing, 211
research toolkit, 122
transitional care, 178

American Nurses Credentialing Center
(ANCC), 204, 213
ANA. *See* American Nurses Association
ANCC. *See* American Nurses
Credentialing Center
animal therapy program, 117
AOCNS. *See* advanced oncology clinical
nurse specialist
APRNs. *See* advanced practice
registered nurses

baccalaureate nursing program, 121
Basic Life Support certificate, 230
behavior-based interviews, 6
questions for CNS candidate, 7
Best Practice Information Sheets
(BPIS), 80
blogs, networking, 172–173
blood glucose levels, using
insulin infusion protocol
control chart, 135
BPIS. *See* Best Practice Information
Sheets
bullying behavior, 71

career-focused professional site, 173
caregivers, 89
case manager, 25
catheter-associated urinary tract infection
(CAUTI), 138, 139
CCC. *See* Critical Care Committee
Centers for Medicare and Medicaid
Services (CMS), 220

certification
  certified clinical nurse specialist (CNS)
    certification options, 205
  employer benefits from, 206
  meanings of, 203–204
  and professional organizations, 204–205
  rationale for, 206
  test-taking skills, 207–208
CINAHL database, 79
clinical currency, 110–111
clinical expertise, 99
clinical ladder program, 138
clinical nurse specialists (CNSs), 23, 33,
    34, 55, 105, 115, 129, 131, 137, 140
  active participation in role, 108–112
  acute care, 182
  becoming preceptor, 106–107
  case manager, 25
  clinical currency and flexibility/
    adaptability in, 105
  clinical days, planning of, 110
  clinical expertise and currency, 110–111
  clinical partnership/experience evalua-
    tion, 112–113
  in clinic/hospital setting, 162
  collaboration, 27–28
  committees and projects work, 111
  community agencies, benefits to, 159
  disciplines and roles, 24–26
  education role and supportive respon-
    sibilities, 111
  functions, direct and indirect, 141–143
  health care systems, complexity
    of, 23–24
  initial phone/e-mail contact, 107
  integration into organization, 26–27
  Internet-based resources, 77–82
  interview process, 18
  job description of. See job
    description, CNS
  job negotiation, 3–11
  keys to effective integration, 29–30
  mentoring staff, 97–104
  monthly tracking sheet, 139
  nurse educator, 24–25
  nurse practitioner, 25
  and nursing roles, 35
  orientation program, 18–19
  performance evaluation, 19
  phases of, 106

  practice environment for, 227–235
  professional association
    involvement, 112
  qualifying for reimbursement, 215–224
  quality managers, 25
  reflect on your role as, 3–4
  relationship and goal setting, 107–108
  reporting relationships of, 28–29
  responsibilities and time-management
    strategies, 111–112
  role and expectations framework, 109
  role in evidence-based practice, 119–120
  role in plan development, 181–183
  role in plan implementation, 183–184
  role in systems thinking and leader-
    ship, 184–185
  role in transitional care, 177,179–186
  role of staff nurse to, 49
  role within organization, 26
  secrets for joyful life as, 237–242
  websites for, 80
  working with boss, fundemental
    practices, 36–41
clinical outcomes,
    documentation, 129–136
  blood glucose levels using insulin
    infusion protocol control chart, 135
  clinical nurse specialists, 131
  control charts, 134
  data elements, definition of, 132–134
  nurse-sensitive outcomes, 130
  outcome evaluation plan, 130, 132
  phases, 129–130
  stakeholders, 131
clinical partnership/experience
    evaluation, 112–113
clinical recognition program, 74
CMS. See Centers for Medicare and
    Medicaid Services
CMS-855I form, 218
CNSs. See clinical nurse specialists
coalitions, community, 158
coding
  for outpatient visits, 222
  for reimbursement, 218, 221
collaboration, 219, 238–239
  for networking, 174
collaborative agreement, 231
collaborative practice, 229–230
collegial relationship, 28

committees
  clinical nurse specialist, 111
  groups, 87, 88
communication, 23
  techniques, 71
  transitional care, 183, 185
communities
  families and, 240
  networking within your, 171
community agencies
  CNS benefits, 159
  community benefits, 158–159
  contacting, 162
  getting started, 159–166
  identification of, 161–162
  institution, benefits to, 159
  maintaining collaborative
    relationships, 166
  patients' benefits, 158
  working with, 157, 162–165
    community-based health
      interventions planning, 164–165
    defining issues to address,
      163–164
    developing relationships with, 163
    intervention evaluation, 165
    intervention implementation, 165
community assessments, 164
Community-Based Care Transitions
  Program, 157
community-based health programs,
  158, 159
  components of, 163
community-based models, of transitional
  care, 177
community health promotion
  interventions, 161
concierge medicine versus private pay,
  234–235
confidentiality agreements, 109
CPT codes. See Current Procedural
  Terminology codes
creative deviance, 239
credentialing process, 211–214
  practice agreements, 230–232
credential verification organization
  (CVO), 212
credibility, establishing, 55–59
  demonstrating, 58–59
  relationships, 56–57

staff nurse credible to expert
  credible, 57–58
Critical Care Committee (CCC), 66
critical-thinking skills, 101
Current Procedural Terminology (CPT)
  codes, 219, 221, 234
CVO. See credential verification
  organization

data collection tools, 133
data elements, definition of, 132–134
delegated versus supervised practice,
  228–229
deviance, creative, 239
diagnosis codes, reimbursement, 222
Diagnostic Related Groupings
  (DRGs), 220
difference, appreciation of, 241
direct functions, 141–143
direct patient care, 18
disciplines and roles, 24–25
documentation, groups, 91
DRGs. See Diagnostic Related Groupings

EBP. See evidence-based practice
education, of patient and health care
  providers, 178
effective change agents, 116
electronic incident reporting system, 50
electronic mailing lists, 172
emergency medical systems (EMS), 196
employment opportunities, for
  networking, 175
EMS. See emergency medical systems
entrepreneurial opportunities, for
  networking, 175
evaluation and management (E/M)
  codes, 234
  reimbursement, 221–222
evidence-based nursing care, 26
evidence-based practice (EBP), 97, 115
  checklist for, 123
  clinical nurse specialist role in, 119–120
  getting started, 120–122
  overview, 115–116
  projects, examples of successful, 117–119
  resources, 26, 79–81
evidence-based scorecard, 141

families and communities, 240
feedback, CNS graduate student, 107
fee for service (FFS), 220
FFS. *See* fee for service

generic orientation classes, value
  of, 45–46
group meetings, 92
  attendance at, 94
groups
  agenda of, 90
  chartering, 88–90
  discussion and follow-up, 90–91
  documentation, 91
  environment and setup, 92
  leader responsibilities, 93–94
  member responsibilities, 94–95
  mentoring new group leaders, 95
  purpose of, 88
  revisiting charter, 96
  schedules, 90
  scope, function, and authority of, 90
  securing resources, 92
  types of, 87–88

handheld technology, 81
health and safety issues, 240
health care, 195
  councils, 88
  environments, 23, 29, 239
  organizations, integration into, 30
  speed and complexity of, 178
health care settings, 238
health care systems, complexity of, 23–24
health care transitions, 185
Health Insurance Portability and
  Accountability Act (HIPAA), 173
health professions education (HPE), 189
HIPAA. *See* Health Insurance Portability
  and Accountability Act
hospital-employed CNSs, 222–223
hospital management information systems, 133
hospitals
  "mentoring on the move," 103
  networking within your, 170–171
  orientation, aspects of, 106
HPE. *See* health professions education

impostor phenomenon, 57
incident-to provision, 220
independent practice, 227–228
independent practitioner, 227
indirect CNS functions, 141–143
industry, networking with, 174
informal mentoring, 74
Institute for Healthcare Improvement
  (2015) website, 78
Institute of Medicine (IOM),
  competencies, 189
insurance reimbursement versus
  Medicare/Medicaid, 234
intellectual power, 153
interdisciplinary collaboration, 23
internal review board (IRB), 144
institutional review board (IRB), 144
International Classification of Diseases
  codes, 222
International Classification of Diseases,
  9th edition (ICD-9), 219
International Classification of Diseases,
  10th edition (ICD-10), 219
Internet-based provider enrolment,
  chain, and ownership system, 218
Internet-based resources
  evidence-based practice resources, 79–81
  handheld technology, 81
  Listservs, 82
  networking, 172
  organizational resources, 78–79
  social media and discussion forums, 81–82
  specialty resources, 81
interprofessional collaborative practice
  (IPCP), 190–195
  competency domains and competen-
    cies, 192–194
  development for, 190
  principles and domains of, 191
interprofessional education (IPE), 189,
    195–197
  CNS participation in, 195
  development for IPCP, 190
  involvement in, 197–198
interprofessional education collaborative
  (IPEC), 195–197
intervention planning, 164
  evaluation of, 165
  implementation of, 165
  summative evaluation, 165

interview process
  preparation for, 6–9, 18
investigating strategies, 117
IPCP. *See* interprofessional
      collaborative practice
IPE. *See* interprofessional education
IPEC. *See* interprofessional education
      collaborative

Joanna Briggs Institute (JBI) website, 80
job description, CNS
  components of, 14–16
  controversies and practical
        solutions, 16–17
  creating, 13–14
  desired qualifications, 16
  to develop CNS tools, 17–19
  position summaries, 14
  principal duties and responsibilities, 14
  required qualifications section, 15
  skills and abilities portion of, 15–16
job offers
  negotiation of, 9–11
  thinking it over, 11
job search, preparation for, 3–4

leaders, 94
  responsibilities, 93–94
life issues, 4–5
life-long learning, 237–238
life/work balance, 64–65
Likert scale, 117–118
LinkedIn, 82, 173
Listservs, 82, 172

Magnet organizations, 70
managed care organizations (MCOs), 211
meaningful evaluation metrics, 119
media-sharing site, 173
Medicaid, 216–217
  versus insurance reimbursement, 234
Medicare, 216
  beneficiaries, 157
  enrollment in, 218
  versus insurance reimbursement, 234
  qualifications, coverage requirements,
        billing, and payment for, 217–218

Medicare Advantage, 216
Medicare Physician Fee Schedule, 217
mentee, 72, 73
mentoring
  definition of, 97–98
  essential qualities for mentor, 98–100
  misconceptions, 101–102
  perspective development, 98
  plan, development of, 100–101
mentoring lens, 70
mentoring mentality, 70
mentoring momentum, 70
"mentoring on the move," 103
mentoring opportunities
  for networking, 174
"mentor intelligence," 70
mentors, 69–76
  benefit of, 73–74
  characteristics of, 70
  collegial and organizational support, 74
  essential qualities for, 98–100
  and mentoring relationships, 70–72
  professional growth, 72–73
  role of, 69
misconceptions, mentoring, 101–102
multidisciplinary rounding team, 88, 90
mutual respect, 196

NACNS. *See* National Association of
      Clinical Nurse Specialists
narrative-reporting format, 140
National Association of Clinical Nurse
      Specialists (NACNS), 14, 177, 205
National Association of Clinical Nurse
      Specialists Listserv (NACNS-list-
      owner@mail-list.com), 82
national CNS core competencies, 13
National Committee for Quality
      Assurance (NCQA), 211
national core competencies, 13
National Council of State Boards of
      Nursing (NCSBN), independent
      practice, 228
National Practitioner Data Bank
      (NPDB), 212
national provider identification (NPI), 218
national provider identifier (NPI), 228
NCQA. *See* National Committee for
      Quality Assurance

networking, 162, 169
  benefits of, 174–175
  on broader scale, 171–174
  with industry, 174
  professional organization, 152
  within your hospital/system, 170–171
  within your local community, 171
"no independent prescribing," 229
"novice-to-expert" approach, 72
NPDB. *See* National Practitioner
  Data Bank
NPI. *See* national provider identification;
  national provider identifier
nurse educators, 24–25
nurse manager, relationship with, 52
nurse practice act, 212
nurse practitioner (NP), 25
nurse-sensitive outcomes, 130
nurse-to-nurse mentoring
  environment, 105
Nursing Model, 213
nursing/nursing practice, 18
  orientation, aspects of, 106
nursing roles, clinical nurse specialist
  and, 35
nursing staff, 62–63
nurturing staff, 99

obstetric hemorrhage algorithm, 118
Omnibus Budget Reconciliation Act of
  1989, 215
Omnibus Reconciliation Act of 1987, 228
Oncology Nursing Certification
  Corporation, 204
Oncology Nursing Society, 206
"oral" portfolio, 4
organizational readiness, 106
organizational resources, 78–79
organization-system category, 141
orientation program, CNS, 18–19
outcome evaluation planning process,
  130, 132
outcomes, internal reporting of, 143–144

PAA. *See* prescriptive authority
  agreement
partnerships, 178, 184
patient-centered care, 195

Patient Protection and Affordable Care
  Act, 189
patient safety committee, 88
PCP. *See* primary care provider
PECOS. *See* provider enrollment, chain,
  and ownership system
pediatric nurse practitioner (PNP), 231
peer group, meeting with, 10
peer review, practice agreements, 232
performance evaluation, 16
  CNS, 19
performance expectations, 138
performance improvement plan, 135
personal credibility, 55
PFS. *See* Physician Fee Schedule
pharmacy systems, 133
Physician Fee Schedule (PFS), Medicare,
  217, 223
physician services, 233, 234
PNP. *See* pediatric nurse practitioner
political power, 153
portfolio, 208
  preparation of, 4
positive mentors, description of, 70–71
positive personal relationship, 100
post-discharge care, 157
PPS. *See* Prospective Payment System
practice
  agreements
    credentialing, 230–231
    protocols, 231
    quality assurance and peer review, 232
  reimbursement
    concierge medicine versus private
     pay, 234–235
    Medicare/Medicaid versus insurance
     reimbursement, 234
    salary versus subcontracting, 232–233
  types of
    collaborative practice, 229–230
    independent practice, 227–228
    supervised versus delegated practice,
     228–229
practice innovations, external reporting
  of, 144–145
prescriptive authority agreement
  (PAA), 231
primary care provider (PCP), 182–183
private pay versus concierge medicine,
  234–235

privileging process, 211–214
professional certification, 206
professional contacts, strong and diverse
    network of, 52
professional development, opportunities
    for, 152–153
professional licensure, 203
professional nursing organization, 15
professional organizations
    certification and, 204–205
    choosing, 149–151
    contribution to profession, 153–154
    getting started, 154
    involvement in, 149
    membership and involvement, benefits
        of, 151–155
    networking, 152
    potential membership benefits, 151
    professional development opportuni-
        ties, 152–153
    providing information, 151–152
    role model for staff, 153
    volunteering, 154–155
    websites, 151
profession, investment in, 239–240
Prospective Payment System (PPS), 220
protocols, practice agreements, 231
provider enrollment, chain, and owner-
    ship system (PECOS), 218
public agencies, 162
PubMed, 79, 81

quality assurance practice
    agreements, 232
quality improvement projects, 144
quality liaison, 25
quality managers, 25

RBRVS. *See* Resource-Based-Relative-
    Value Scale
Recovery and Reinvestment Act, 189
reflection, reserve time for, 52–53
registered nurse (RN), 99
reimbursement
    coding for, 218, 221
        outpatient visits, 222
    CPT codes, 221
    diagnosis codes, 222

evaluation and management codes,
    221–222
hospital-employed CNSs, 222–223
legislation background, 215–216
Medicaid, 216–217
Medicare, 216
    enrollment in, 218
    qualifications, coverage
        requirements, billing, and
        payment for, 217–218
practice
    concierge medicine versus private
        pay, 234–235
    Medicare/Medicaid versus insurance
        reimbursement, 234
    salary versus subcontracting, 232–233
productivity track, 223
terms used, 219
third-party reimbursement entities, 216
relationship-building values, 197
relative-value unit (RVU), 219
research
    APRN regulations, 6
    of employer, 5
    state licensure requirements, 5–6
Resource-Based-Relative-Value Scale
    (RBRVS), 219
responsibilities, clinical nurse
    specialists, 111–112
risk management systems, 133
RN. *See* registered nurse
role ambiguity, avoiding, 49–51
roles and disciplines, CNS, 24–26
role socialization, 73
RVU. *See* relative-value unit

salary versus subcontracting, 232–233
scorecards
    CNS, 140
    creating, 140–143
service opportunities, for networking, 172
shared values, 196
SMART goals, 51
social media, 173
    and discussion forums, 81–82
    opportunities, for networking, 172
Social Security Act of 1965, 216
sounding board, acting as, 100
specialty certification, 206, 208

specialty organizations, 81
specialty resources, 81
SRL. *See* systematic reviews of the
    literature
staff nurse to CNS, role of, 49
stakeholders, 131
Statement on Clinical Nurse Specialist
    Practice and Education, 15
structured recording tool, 18
subcommittee, 88
subcontracting versus salary, 232–233
summative evaluation, intervention, 165
supervised versus delegated practice,
    228–229
supervision, types of, 35–36
sustainable transition care programs, 159
systematic reviews of the literature
    (SRL), 80

task groups, 87
teaching, 100
team dynamics, principles of, 197
test-taking skills, 207–208
The Joint Commission (TJC), 211, 212
third-party reimbursement entities, 216
"three spheres of influence," 14
time management, 61, 64
    strategies for, 111–112
toxic mentors, 71
tracking sheet, 139–140
transitional care
    challenge in, 184
    CNS role in, 179–186

community-based models of, 177
    elements of, 178–179
    health care transitions, 185
    patient-centered plan for, 185
tweets, 82
Twitter, 81–82, 173

virtual mentoring, 101
volunteering
    professional organizations, 154–155
    for projects, 170

web-based discussion forums, 82
websites
    for clinical nurse specialist, 80
    Joanna Briggs Institute, 80
    National Association of Clinical Nurse
        Specialists, 177
    professional organizations, 151
work groups, formation of, 92
worksheets, 138–139
WPA. *See* written practice agreement
"written" portfolio, 4
written practice agreement (WPA),
    230, 231

YouTube, 173

Printed in the United States
By Bookmasters